Dr Nic Andela

Dissecting Humour

Burgundy
publishing

A Burgundy Publishing Book

Published by Burgundy Publishing South Africa 2005

The moral right of the author has been asserted.

A CIP catalogue record of this book is available from the British
Library and the State Library in South Africa.

ISBN 0 9551 2680 0

Printed and bound in South Africa by Print Ability

Burgundy Publishing cc
322 Rivonia Boulevard, Rivonia, Gauteng
P O Box 2114, Randburg, 2125, South Africa

Burgundy
publishing

Preface

Infections, depression, stress, cancer and its gruelling treatments, spinal injuries, war, cultural intolerance, relationship decay and emotional pain seem to involve more and more people we know. How often do we find ourselves sinking into despair, contemplating the realities and complexities of today's living?

Recently, my mother developed mouth floor cancer. As a consequence, she received invasive neck clearance surgery, and immediately thereafter developed dire post-operative intensive care complications. She was then subjected to months of radiotherapy, and is now very weak. She is now in remission but is suffering from depression. In spite of all these necessary but dreadful interventions, she maintains a joyful sense of humour.

I dedicate this book to her; as well as to anyone who is suffering from cancer, experiencing anxiety, and is finding it difficult to cope.

Humour has healing properties. It can generate pleasure at any moment. It can reboot your mind, so that you can appreciate the things you have around you but temporarily forget about. Humour crosses cultural boundaries, reducing stress and tension.

To my co-author, Janine, and the illustration team, Ilana and Judith, who worked many late hours outside of their regular jobs to produce and complete Dissecting Humour Volume 1, thank you for all your hard work.

Many thanks to Audrey Cooper for your endless support and input. Thanks to all the staff at LBH for putting up with me for the last three years.

And finally my publisher, Liz Jones of Burgundy Publishing, I thank you for your support, your time and for having enough faith to take this project forwards and also Symoné-Leigh for the design and layout.

Dissecting Humour is filled with supposed urban legends. I hope that these stories help you to escape from reality, and that you allow this bizarre humour and laughter to gain new perspective on your life.

Contents

Adrenalin Med-Student Drinkers

A six-year medical curriculum is challenging. A medical student has to find time for hospital ward rounds, theatre lists and patient clinics. All in addition, lectures for the vast number of academic subjects covered simultaneously. It is this combination that sets the medical course apart from other professional courses.

I remember preparing, at two-thirty, one Friday morning, for a second year anatomical exam. I still had mountains of material to work through. The exam started at eight-thirty in the morning.

Tiredness set in. I decided to set my alarm to wake me at five o'clock, dragging me out of a deep sleep. Drinking one of the strongest cups of coffee ever created, I continued with my studies. My hands propping my head up, I desperately tried to keep my eyes focused. Why was I so tired? This routine was nothing new. Being a morning-person, those few hours usually did me a great service. I peered down at my wristwatch and saw that it was only three-thirty! The alarm clock must have been on the blink. Bugger it! I jumped back into bed and slept until eight o'clock. Sure, I'd have to thumb-suck a little but at least I had my lucky quartz crystal – everything would be fine.

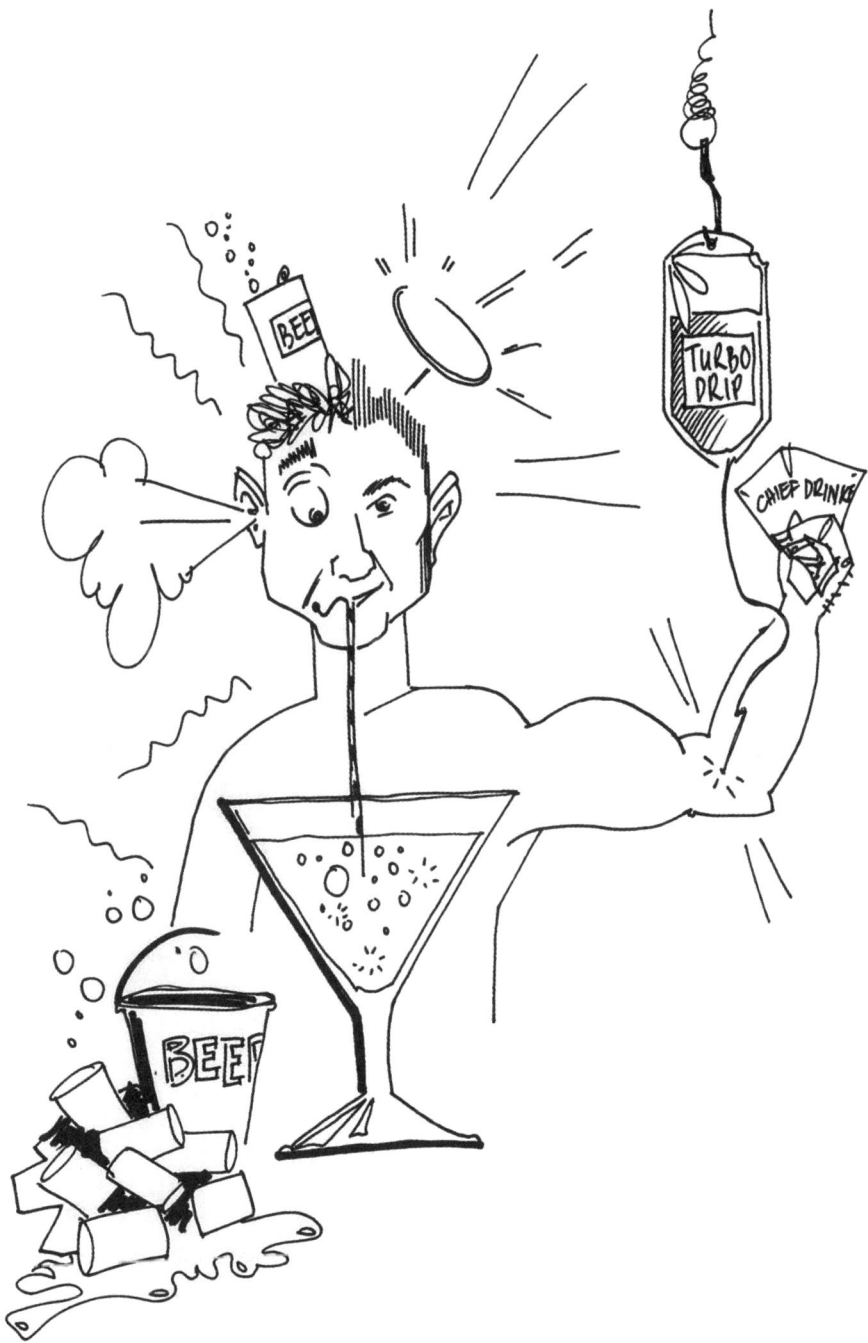

3

That pattern of late nights and early mornings is an integral part of life as a med-student, and lasts the full six years. So how do med-students manage to keep up their collective reputation for being party animals? Could it be all the coffee consumed during training, which increases the cytochromic liver enzymes and therefore metabolism? Could it simply be a determination to express social freedom, as much as other students do; out on the piss more than four days out of the seven?

I'll tell you something right now. It's neither. Medical science has all the answers.

We medics were in digs together, sharing a commune for three years before moving on. The Bradley twins were a pair of rascals. Their red Ford 4x4 pick-up with frightening petrol consumption of about one gallon per ten miles was their run-around. I remember several occasions when they stole petrol from parked cars on the campus. Wide rims, Yokohama tyres and a double cab; we named the pick-up 'Bruce.' What a babe-magnet the Bruce was.

Simon Bradley bought the Bruce cheap. Aunt Molly left him money after her sad demise, following a hit-and-run accident. Though she had no way of knowing it, Aunt Molly was partly responsible for putting us on the university map.

We were inseparable, especially during social hours at big student bashes. We weren't sporting legends or campus jocks. Although we were caring, diligent and focused medical students, we needed to find our niche within the campus hierarchy. We could be spotted from a mile off at a social, just by looking at our glasses of mix. There would always be a couple of the pre-injection gauze alcohol Sterets that doctors use to clean the skin, floating on the surface. We became the 'Drinking Legends'!

There was no one on campus who could out-drink us. Not even the seven-foot monster-men, or the pre-alcoholic law students. It was amusing to see how our lean five-foot-seven frames could intimidate those who considered themselves to be big men. We always felt superior as we stepped over the bodies covering the floor, making our haughty exit at the end of a particularly raucous party.

The secret was in the backs of our hands and in the back of the Bruce.

A hangover is the result of ethanol consumption. Ethanol is a diuretic that causes excessive urination, depleting your intrinsic water capacity. Alcohol metabolism in the liver leads to the production of an aldehyde derivative. The accumulation of this by-product is responsible for the effects of a hangover, significantly increased by dehydration. Alcohol metabolism is also responsible for hypoglycaemia - low glucose levels, gastric irritation and heartburn.

Medical school and pharmacology helped us transform the acute alcohol treatment regime into our own alcohol resistance regime!

I laugh whenever I think back to the Medical Ball. A limited number of tickets were allocated. The theme was "pink". The party committee had leased an old farmhouse for the night. More than three hundred partygoers attended it, all making full use of the bar that offered only one type of beer on tap. A couple of hundred hay bales offered a farmyard atmosphere, and a live band provided the music.

When we arrived at eight-thirty, the party was in full swing. There were around a hundred cars parked in the vicinity. We noticed Mike Daniels, a law student who could drink with the big boys. There were many occasions when he may have endangered his life trying to keep up with us, blissfully unaware that we had an alcohol resistance regime.

Before any party we would prepare at the digs. Working at hospitals gave us access to the one litre ten percent glucose drips, drip sets, H2 antagonists (heartburn and gastric irritation drugs) and a vitamin B combination. Mix the H2 and Vitamin B complex together in a litre bag of glucose, which then turns yellow. You then have the perfect acute alcohol treatment regime, which also translates as the perfect alcohol resistance regime!

Bradley had inserted ten drip-holder hooks into the ceiling of the Bruce. On the night of the Pink Party we had ten prepared bags and drip sets on the hooks – ready for action! We inserted venflons intravenously into the backs of our hands and secured them with clinical tape, which would be concealed by our party clothes.

The drinking began. We socialised with fellow students that we knew, others that we would know by the end of the night. The evening progressed and whenever one of us would feel a little bleak and intoxicated, the plan would kick in.

Excusing himself for a bathroom break, Byron disappeared into the back of the Bruce, shut the door and rolled up his sleeve to expose the drip site. He then hooked up to the drip line, lay down for five minutes and let the drip do its work before returning - very much refreshed - to the party. The rest of us followed the routine as and when necessary.

Admittedly, it took a while before we decided it would be prudent to pre-mix the bags at the beginning of the evening. You don't need to be pissed whilst trying to aspirate drugs and inject them into drip bags using sharp needles, at two in the morning. We found that it got bloody and messy.

Once we had perfected the technique, those bags took us through the evening and carried us on to the early hours. We were victorious! Party after party, we were always the last men standing.

Safari Ambulance

Ben and Koffie were paramedics tasked with covering the wide-spread third world district of northern Thula, on a salary that wouldn't give them half an hour's shopping time on Sloane Street. This depressing reality meant that they wouldn't pass up any opportunity that came their way.

In the very early hours one morning, they were bumping along a dirt track on their way back to the decrepit ambulance station. Koffie hit the brakes to avoid a large male Kudu, lying in the road. Turning on the spotlights, they got out to investigate.

The antelope had probably been hit by a truck that passed along the road a while earlier. The animal's spirit had departed, leaving behind a beautiful lean body glazed with streaks of blood. Its horns were magnificent, thick and long, with at least four spirals each.

Ben and Koffie looked at each other. The carcass could feed a number of their immediate family and friends for at least a week. "What are we waiting for?" Ben asked. They went to the back of the ambulance, and removed the spinal board, six rolls of elastoplast strapping, the patient-trolley and two carrier poles. The antelope was well-lit, but beyond the beam of the spotlights, the night was like a black curtain.

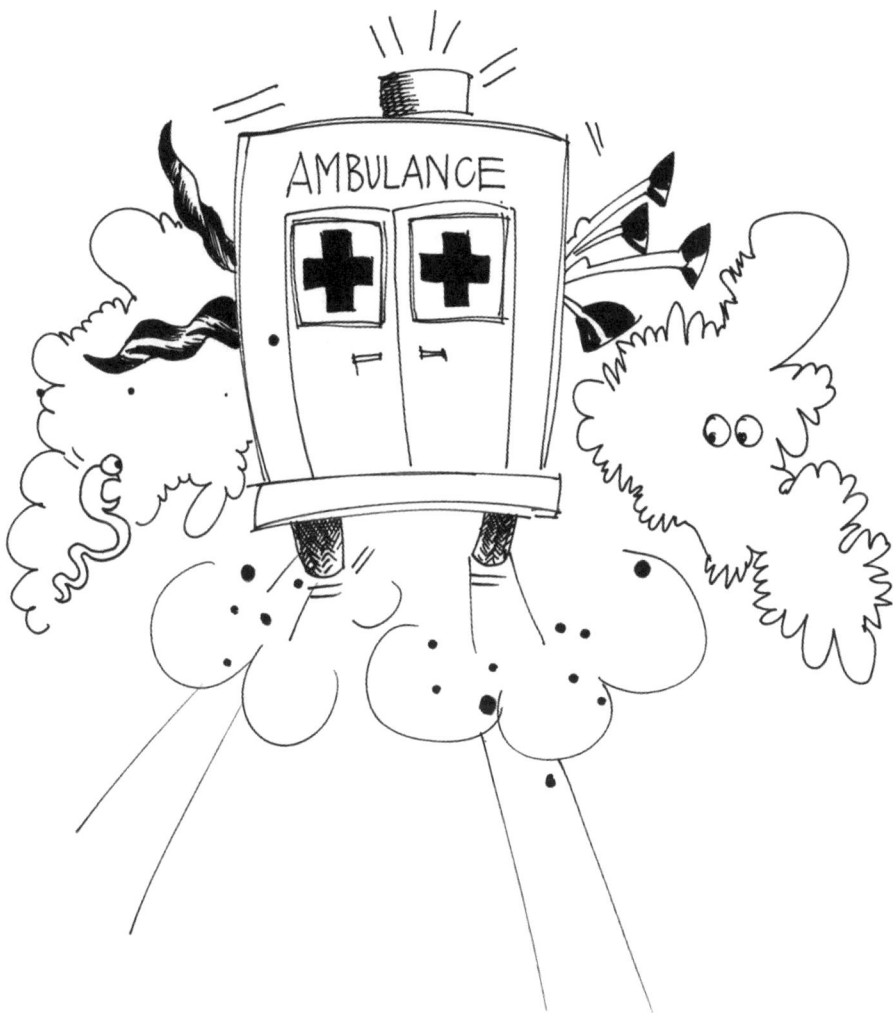

Working swiftly to the tune of the usual nocturnal insect orchestra, Ben and Koffie managed to get the antelope strapped firmly to the spinal board. The strapping paramedics nearly buckled under the weight of the carcass. With a mixture of determination and profanity, they managed to lift it onto the trolley, and then slide it into the ambulance. In order to get the doors closed, Koffie had to hop in and open the windows, so that the horns stuck out of one side of the vehicle, and the legs out of the other. The body itself really didn't take up much room at all.

They were barely back on their way, when a call came through that a confused granny with Alzheimer's had fallen and injured her hip. The paramedics were required to pick her up, and transport her to the small local hospital. Tutting loudly, Koffie put his foot to the floor. As they reached busier roads, Ben flicked on the flashing blue light and faulty siren. It must have been quite a sight: the ambulance zipping through the streets, lights flashing, siren wailing and hiccupping, hooves and horns protruding from the windows!

When they got to the granny's address she was sitting outside, in her nightgown, regaling all who stopped to listen with stories of the good old days. "Ah! Here's my taxi!" she cackled as Ben and Koffie pulled up. They managed to wedge her into the ambulance, squeezed between the antelope's rump and a large oxygen bottle. She didn't seem to notice that her travelling companion didn't have much to say. Koffie fed the drip line through the window, and hung the vaculiter drip on one of the antelope's horns.

As he slammed the doors closed, Ben shouted, "Hold tight! We'll get you to the hospital in no time!"

Minutes later, Granny was being pried out of the tight corner of the ambulance and wheeled, on a trolley, into hospital. "We always get out patients here safely," Koffie boasted.

"Well, I don't know about that other one," Granny whispered, pointing a gnarled finger over her shoulder at the ambulance. "He didn't seem very well at all!"

Suicide Dash

An academic hospital during dark African nights can be a very cold and lonely place. Only the casualty department, delivery suites and operating theatres seem to hum with activity, and their own particular bloody smells. The other wards are characterised by quietness and darkness, accommodating both sleeping patients and some exhausted staff.

Most of the hospitals have long, dirty corridors, branching off to numerous wards. Look carefully, and you might see a cockroach or two scuttling into the cracks in the floor. People tend to walk briskly past them, hurrying to escape the eerie feeling of being watched by unseen eyes.

The weekend's ritualistic hustle and bustle of the casualty department, filled with violently injured patients, has the potential to drive doctors away. If you were a doctor on such a night, and you were suddenly presented with an opportunity to have the night off, would you need to think twice before grabbing it with both hands? I didn't think so!

Three medical officers were given this golden opportunity one evening, due to a mix up with the anaesthetic rota. Two of them were free to leave. Unfortunately, all three doctors were stubborn, unaccommodating and utterly inflexible. A conflict of interests arose. Which two would go? Who would stay to complete the shift?

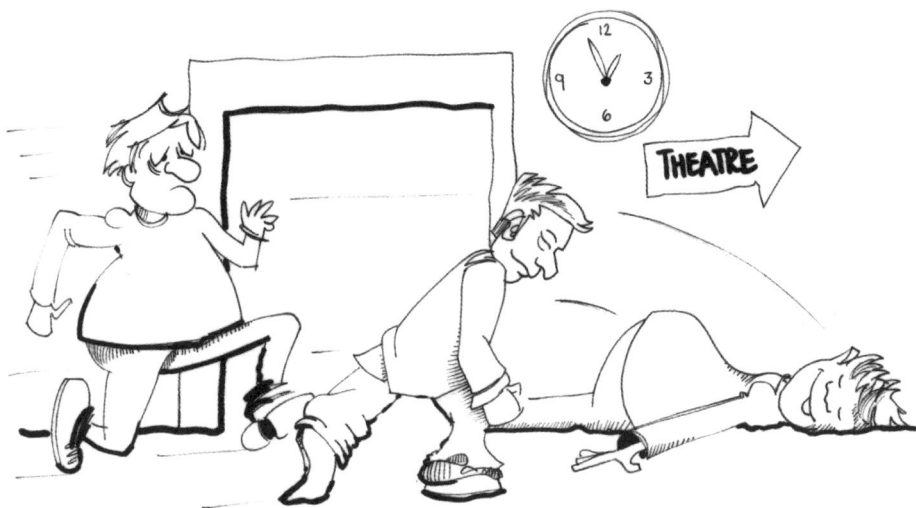

It was one o'clock in the morning when they received the splendid news of the rota cock-up. Given their odd hours and elevated adrenalin levels, these shift doctors could be forgiven for irrational thought processes. Who knew what solution they would think up?

Scholine is a cheap anaesthetic drug, used by doctors throughout the world to temporarily paralyse a patient needing to be operated on. As you can well imagine, anxiety levels tend to soar in a conscious patient who finds himself on an operating table, unable to move a muscle- let alone breathe- while doctors hover around, holding sharp scalpels and other scary-looking surgical equipment. That is why it is considered good medical practice to give a patient a simultaneous dose of a sleeping drug. What you don't know won't hurt you, as they say!

Since Scholine is a muscle relaxant, it will paralyse the breathing muscles. It is therefore essential that a patient is intubated. This involves inserting a breathing tube through the patient's nose or mouth, sliding it through the voice box so that it comes to rest in the trachea. The other end of the tube is fixed to either a mechanical breathing machine, or a manually operated ambu bag to maintain a normal oxygen concentration within the patient's lungs.

The bottom line is this: Do not allow anyone to give you a dose of Scholine without first ensuring that someone trustworthy is on hand to breathe for you. Suffocation is not a pleasant way to exit!

Our three courageous doctors trusted each other implicitly. This is a good thing, given the unorthodox manner in which they would solve their dilemma.

A corridor with a length in excess of a hundred metres was the chosen venue for the appropriately named "Suicide Dash." They kicked off the proceedings by inserting a plastic sheath, called a cannula, into the back of each others' hands to allow quick access to a vein for later administration of drugs. They had the good sense to arrange the necessary resuscitation equipment from a nearby emergency trolley: intubation equipment, resuscitation drugs, an oxygen cylinder and an ambu bag.

One at a time, a fixed dose of Scholine was given through the cannula. The drugged doctor then ran as far as possible down the corridor before he collapsed from the paralysing effects of the drug.

He was then entirely dependent on his two colleagues to breathe for him for about five minutes, when the effects would wear off. The spot where the doctor had fallen was marked with chalk. Then another doctor would take a turn. The two doctors who managed to run the furthest were relieved of the burden of the graveyard shift.

It is amazing what extreme sports some people will take part in just to get a night off work!

Bedside Manners

Ward rounds are an everyday occurrence in hospitals all over the world. They constitute a vital part of the treatment process. Medical information filters down a hierarchy; from the professor to the most junior doctor. The rounds are characterised by groups of doctors wearing white coats that flutter behind them like super heroes' capes, as they move briskly from bedside to bedside. These bedside congregations result in discussions, instructions and most importantly, health care decisions.

I have always wondered how in-patients feel when a group descends upon them, when they are at their most vulnerable. Do they feel intimidated? Scared? Relieved or embarrassed? Would you like to have your haemorrhoids discussed by a group of trainees, as you lay in bed with nowhere to hide your blushes?

From early on in medical school, our senior peers emphasise the need to respect our patients, empathise with their problems, and to behave in a professional manner at all times. Our bedside manners will determine how popular we are with patients and staff alike.

Professor Mathers was a well-respected surgeon whose results in the operating room spoke for themselves. His bedside manner, however, left a lot to be desired. His reputation was well known among the junior doctors.

One day, our group arrived at the bedside of Mrs McKenna; an overweight, middle aged woman who had struggled for years with her knees. Osteoarthritis and severe bone degeneration of the knee

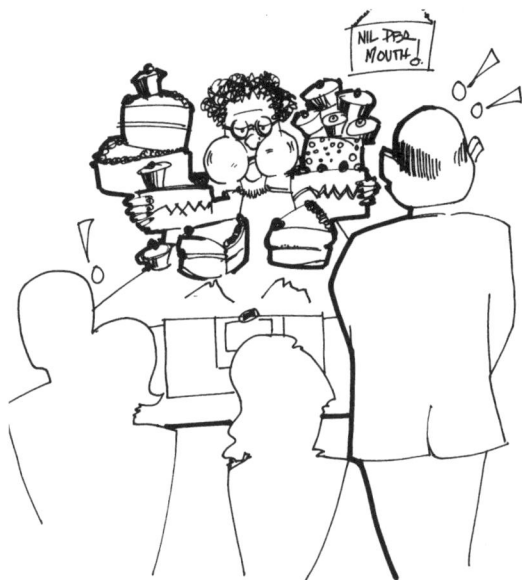

joints had caused pain and limited movement. Despite her recent knee replacement, she remained painfully loud, though optimistic.

We all crowded around, with Professor 'Bedside Bad Manners' taking up position at the foot of the bed. He was already utterly frustrated by the fact that Mrs McKenna had been less than cooperative with her pre-op diet program. The cakes and sweets piled high on her bedside table did nothing to improve his mood.

You could have heard a surgical pin drop, as the Professor muttered rudely, "Madam, you eat far too much, and that is why your knees have packed up!"

"Oh but Doctor," Mrs McKenna protested, "I only eat like a little bird!"

"What!" Professor barked. "Lady, you eat more like a greedy vulture!"

And with that statement hanging in the air, the Professor stormed out of the room, leaving everyone, including the hapless patient, quite flabbergasted.

Car-Jacking

Sam Naiad had flown into Cape Town from the sunny coast of Durban. He sat in a cab on the highway, waiting for the congestion to clear so he could get moving again. He was excited about seeing his relative, but couldn't help remembering the anxious faces of his wife and three kids as he said goodbye at the airport that morning. The Cape had been in a state of high alert, after a string of recent car-jackings.

Mabulubizi was nineteen and alone. His parents had died of AIDS, and his grandmother had been too financially stretched and old to take care of the young orphan. She died of a stroke soon afterwards, leaving Mabulubizi with no choice, but to develop a bucket load of street sense and independence. Schooling had never been an option, as it didn't bring in cash, and, anyway, neither school nor the tattered local social services would be able to help him.

Tragically, this is not an uncommon scenario, and is played out throughout the world, with no hope of changing any time soon.

Mabulubizi was driven, by poverty and circumstance, into crime. He had killed before, during a car jacking, and would do so again for the couple of thousand rands he received per unit. The gun fired, and the middle-aged woman was flung backwards into the street. Mabulubizi sped off in her BMW. Luckily the bullet missed all her major organs. This particular victim of violent crime would live to tell the tale.

Mabulubizi felt nothing. He was past any form of rehabilitation.

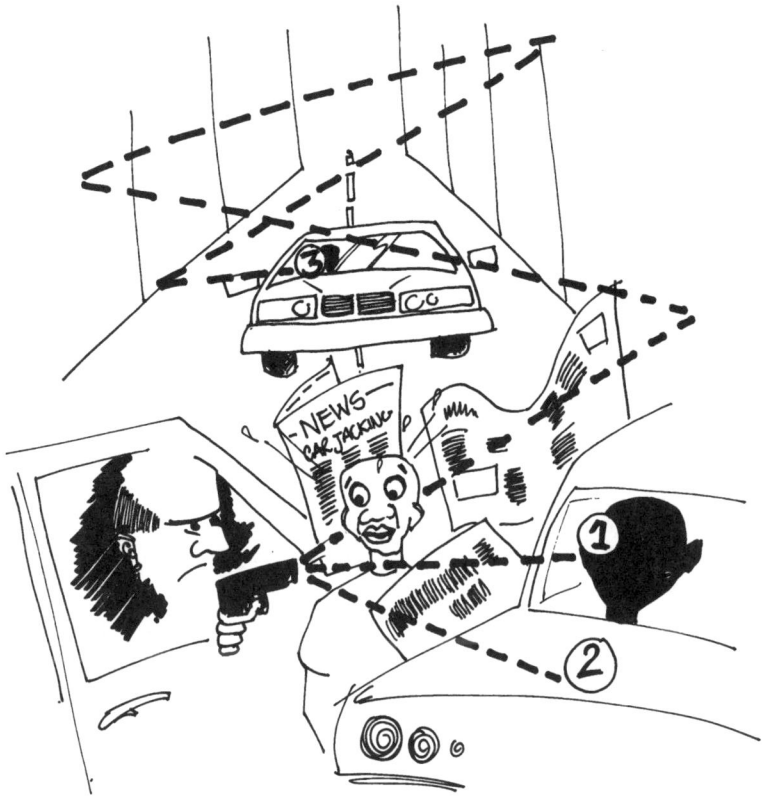

Murray had been in the paramedic service for five years. He had seen some grim sights in that time. Just the other day, he and Matt had been called to an accident on the highway. A car driving at about seventy miles per hour had hit a pedestrian. On arriving at the scene, they found a large area of the road covered in blood, flesh and limbs that had been ripped off by the impact. Fingers were wedged into the front windscreen and wiper blades. Both lower limbs had been forced upwards by the huge forces involved. The corpse lay chest down, and the two femur hip balls protruded through the victim's buttocks. The articular surfaces were clean and shiny. Pieces of flesh coating the femur were all that was left of the muscles. The police eventually found the victim's capitum, or what was left of the head, about one hundred and fifty yards from the crash site.

This type of climate is far from ideal for some. Ray Jennings, an ex-Special Forces lieutenant, practised shooting once a week at the local shooting range. He had maintained his small arms skills after he had left the corps. His time of special operations in small, congested township environments, had taken its toll on Ray. The dangerous missions, and the colleagues who had died in his arms, had resulted in post-traumatic syndrome. Therapy played a positive role in Ray's rehabilitation. However, reading about violent acts, as reported in the media, didn't help. He began to carry his side arm wherever he went: in the supermarket, in the car, and even at home.

Thando was a child of the streets. Thirteen years old, with no father, and little interaction with his mother. The lack of proper role models led to him forming alliances with other street kids. Life had been cruel to these innocents, and they looked for an avenue of escape. A few cents would buy the gang a small paint tin of cheap industrial glue, and the world could be blotted out for a while. Petty crime would pay for the next fix. Thando reached a point where he had to make a major life decision: the gang and its ways, or his job, selling newspapers at a popular traffic light intersection.

A few days previously, Ray had picked up the newspaper, and had seen pictures of the woman who had been thrown from her BMW during a car jacking. He was outraged. He told himself, "Just let them try...I'll give them a bit of the lead stuff!" He gripped his revolver tightly.

Now he sat stationary in the traffic jam, reading the paper as he waited for the cars in front to move.

Sam sat next to the cab driver, sweltering in the heat. They edged onto the off-ramp, and moved slowly towards the intersection. Sam couldn't wait to get to his air-conditioned hotel.

Thando could see a man reading the morning newspaper in his car. Maybe this was a good opportunity to sell him the afternoon edition. He rushed off towards the vehicle before the traffic moved. Out of the corner of his eye, Ray could see a figure coming towards him and sat bolt upright.

"No you don't, you motherf*****!" He ripped the revolver out of its holster, and fired through the door. Bang! Bang! Bang! The shot rang out and Thando got the fright of his life. He threw the papers into the air and screamed.

In the cab, Sam felt a burning pain in his thigh and cried out. There were two holes in the side of the cab, and blood everywhere. The cab driver was stunned, and fumbled for the mike to radio his control centre. Stammering, he managed to describe what had happened, and control sent for an ambulance.

Through the roiling gun smoke and ringing in his ears, Ray noticed Thando lying in the street between his car and Sam's cab.

"What have I done?" he sobbed. He looked out, despairingly, for a couple of seconds, before flinging his revolver aside, and going to help.

Murray was speechless when he arrived on the scene. Traffic was backed up for a couple of miles. A boy with a flesh wound to his inner thigh lay screaming, possibly with relief that his ding-dong was still where it should be, amongst a pile of newspapers. Another man was sitting in a cab, clutching his thigh. A pale, clueless man, dashed between the two, being of no help to either.

Matt called out, "Murray, we've just got another call! Some guy a block away took a head shot through the windscreen. Apparently, he was driving a stolen Beamer!"

Morgue Prankster

Rob Barns is an eligible bachelor who recently turned thirty-three. After completing his medical degree, he decided to specialise in a career in Forensic Anatomical Pathology, at Luke's General University Hospital. These are the guys who examine human bodies, to make assessments according to macroscopic, microscopic and dissection findings. He is now a full-time specialist and lecturer at Luke's.

It is an interesting field of work. When a dead body is found, forensic medicine allows the scientist to estimate the time of death, by studying the life cycle stages of parasitic worms found in the body. It doesn't sound too pleasant; but it gives the police a focal point for their investigations.

The Anatomical Department accepts one or two postgraduates a year, depending on the funding available. Rob has a reputation for introducing the new doctors to the department, with a short speech and a tour of the facilities.

Rob performed his usual routine for Jeff Fields and Di Watson. He marched them into the laboratories, showing them the microscopes and electron microscopes. He assured them that they would soon be as familiar with these instruments, as they were with their own mobile phones.

"I have a surprise for you!" Rob announced with a smile. "We have a fresh one here today – just came in!"
"What did?" Di looked confused. "John Smith: our latest corpse," Rob informed her. "The cops brought him in, and requested a full work over. I hear he was shot-up pretty bad!" Rob said, gleefully.

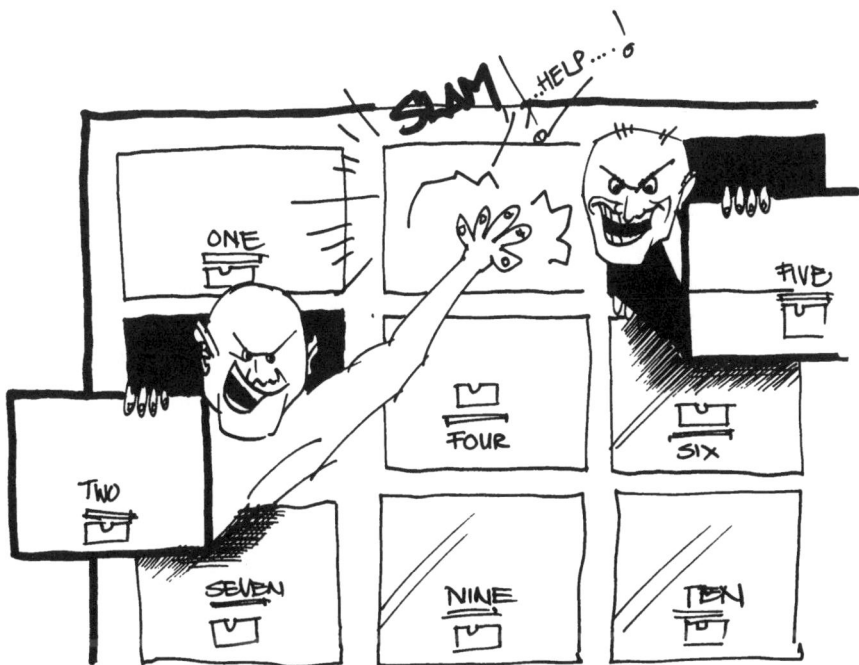

They walked into the dim, eerily quiet dissection room in the morgue. The air felt damp, and there was a faint metallic-chemical smell. A dull rattling noise came from the refrigeration unit. Inside, twenty gurneys were stacked, each on steel runners, allowing them to slide in and out easily. A label on each small door identified the body on the gurney within. In the centre of the room, four steel legs supported a stainless steel table, with a drain at the bottom end and a hosepipe at the top. On the table lay a body, covered with a bloodstained sheet. Every few seconds the drain would gurgle as body fluids escaped from the corpse.

"Guys, this is our bread and butter. This is where we have to perform!" Rob told them. "Please put on these gloves and aprons," he tossed the items at Jeff and Di, "Stand at the side of the table and do the preliminary macroscopic assessments for me." Rob stood back, waiting to be impressed.

Di was anxious, even though she had dissected a corpse in medical school. She slowly peeled back the sheet and exposed the body; facial features were obscured by blood, and the torso oozed a foul-smelling yellow substance.

"Where are the arms?" Jeff wondered aloud from the opposite side of the table. As if to answer the question, a hand shot out of either side of the bloody sheet, grabbed Jeff and Di around the backside and pulled them in towards the table. Di almost screamed the place down. Jeff was struck dumb with fright, grabbing hold of the hosepipe to stop himself from collapsing on the floor in a dead faint. It was seconds before they realised that Rob and the 'corpse' were howling with laughter; Rob doubled up over a counter, and the corpse sitting up, clutching his sides with mirth.

It was some time before everyone had calmed down enough to speak. "I'm really sorry!" Rob said, although he didn't sound anything like it. "It's my little tradition – Welcome to the Luke's Anatomical Department!" He pointed at the 'corpse'. "Meet Jon Denver, a consultant here."

The gag didn't go down very well with the new recruits. Jeff remained nervous for the first year. Di was the type of person who bore a grudge.

Two years later, she suggested that Rob change his traditional gag. "Why don't you get into one of the slots and play dead? When Jon brings the new guys in, he can get them to open the door of the fridge, and you can grab them." Rob agreed that it would be a great wheeze.

On January the seventh, Rob woke up and leapt into the shower. Two new recruits would be starting that morning, and Rob was looking forward to trying out the new prank. Once in the morgue, Jon used some of Di's make-up to give Rob's face and torso a deathly pale appearance. Rob opened the number-five door of the fridge, and sprang onto the gurney. "What time are you bringing them in?" he asked Jon.

"Di will bring them in about twenty minutes – I've got to dash off!" Jon explained. "But it's tradition!" Rob protested.

"Can't be helped!" Jon shouted, as he rushed out of the room.

Sighing, Rob covered himself with a sheet, gripped the sides of the fridge, and thrust himself inside. The gurney slid in smoothly and the door shut, sealing Rob inside the refrigeration unit. It was completely dark. Rob felt the cold in his bones. "Where are they?" he muttered, as his teeth began to chatter. The minutes felt like hours and he started to worry. He tried to push the door open with his feet but it was stuck fast. The hairs on the back of his neck stood up and a chill ran down his spine. "I could die in here! I'm such a knob!" Rob suffered an acute sense-of-humour failure, and started to yell. "Help! Open up! I'm stuuuck!"

In the cold dark fridge, a hand reached out and clutched Rob's forearm tightly, jerking him towards the number-six slot. As Rob screamed in terror, another hand grabbed his ankle and pulled. It felt as if he would be pulled apart! Screaming like a lunatic, Rob tried to thrash his arms and legs, but the space was limited. Just as he was about to lose his mind he heard a snicker.

"What the hell...?" He heard roars of laughter from within the fridge and outside. Suddenly the door opened, and light flooded into the fridge. He could see most members of the department standing in the room, laughing and slapping each other on the back. Two more fridge doors opened, and out slid Jeff and Jon, giggling their heads off.

"You bloody bastards! Are you trying to kill me?" Rob laughed with relief.

"It was all Di's idea," Jon told him. "Not bad, eh?"

Criminal Remorse

1 a.m.

It was Sunday the thirteenth of March. The exchange of gunfire could be heard echoing around the suburb. A few yards away, PC Smith lay motionless in a pool of blood; shot in the chest. Police Constable Graham sustained a bullet wound to the abdomen, and was taken to hospital for treatment. The remaining officers assisted the gun reinforcement unit, who had taken up sniper positions on the flanks of nearby buildings, barricading all possible escape routes from the criminals' dwelling.

An hour beforehand, a motor patrol had reported a suspicious vehicle heading towards the coast on the M3. As the patrol approached the Lexus, its driver accelerated and took the next off-ramp. The pursuit ended in the suburbs. More police units were called to assist in the chase. Shots were fired from the Lexus, leaving one officer fatally wounded. The gun unit was called in immediately.

After a long chase, the Lexus was forced into a cul-de-sac. Five felons, one carrying a large holdall, ran from the car and into a house. Armed with automatic rifles and smaller handguns, a gunfight ensued, in which two felons were killed. The law enforcement agency had accidentally stumbled upon a large-scale drug exchange, and had stopped the perpetrators from reaching their meeting point.

The gunfight continued into the early hours of the morning, when two more felons were shot dead. The gang leader was hit in the chest and stomach. Paramedics were escorted into the house, where the

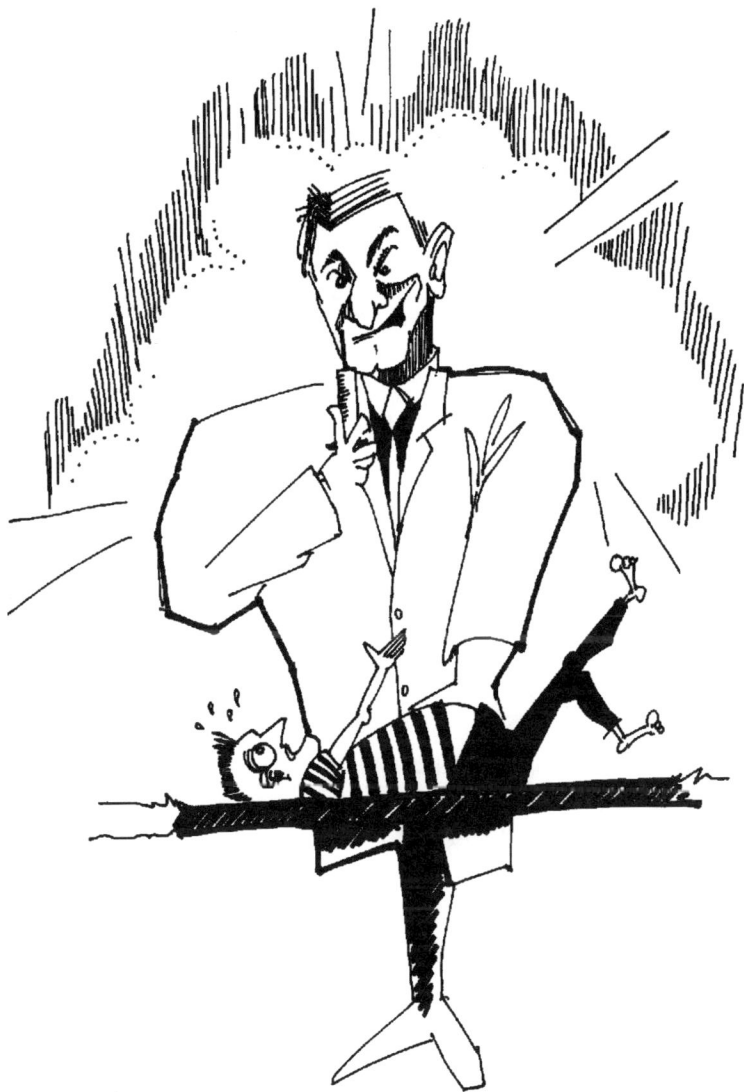

injured felon was resuscitated and taken to the ambulance. The man was a beast. His language was foul, and he thrashed around trying to fight off the paramedics as they attempted to treat him. He was restrained by three PCs, who accompanied him to the hospital.

5 a.m.

It was Dan Summer's last shift on call. Continuous exposure to violent acts and unsatisfactory working conditions had driven him to embrace a new career in business. He was looking forward to regular working hours, and a chance to regain his compassion so that the Hippocratic Oath might, once again, mean something to him. As the injured felon was brought in, Dan was called. An emergency anaesthetic and laparotomy were required. The patient had kept up his uncooperative attitude.

"Doc, we've got a cop killer here! Pity he made it this far!"

"Wonderful!" Dan said through gritted teeth, as the healthcare staff pushed the trolley to the anaesthetic room.

Two PCs stood, armed and ready for trouble, looking around the room, fascinated by all the shiny equipment laid out for the operation. Restraints were used to keep the patient still as he lay on the trolley.

Dan took a deep breath as he entered the room. "Listen, I am your anaesthetist – not the police," he told the patient. "I need to give you an anaesthetic cocktail so you can sleep during the operation on your stomach. First, I will give you a painkiller called Fentanyl and then Propofol to send you to sleep. Once you are asleep, you'll be given Scholine, which will relax all the muscles in your body. A breathing tube will be inserted, and a ventilator will breathe for you. OK?" Dan leaned over the patient.

"You f****** asshole! I wish you would die like those other pigs out there!" The patient ended his short speech by spitting in Dan's face.

Dan grabbed a towel and wiped the green slime from his face. He turned to the policemen and said, in a pleasant but forceful tone, "I would like to congratulate you on the superb work you have done tonight in capturing this man and bringing him here. Can I ask you outstanding gents to wait outside for a minute?"

Unable to decide who was scarier - the Doctor or the patient – the cops left in a hurry.

Dan removed the oxygen mask from the patient, and took the Scholine from the tray. He injected the patient with 300mg, three times the normal dose, and watched closely. The man on the trolley began to twitch violently but a few seconds later he lay still and tranquil, staring into Dan's eyes. He could no longer breathe, talk or move, but he could see, hear and feel.

Dan watched as the patient began to suffocate, becoming cyanotic. His vital signs were going off the chart, with high blood pressure and a very high pulse rate; a grave stress response. The saturation monitor alarmed slower and slower. The oxygen content fell below sixty percent.

Dan grinned humourlessly. "Do you know that you are dying now, and I pretty much own you?" He picked up the ambu bag, applied the oxygen mask to the patient's face, and bagged him a few breaths of one hundred percent oxygen, until the saturation level moved above the ninety percent mark. Then Dan stopped.

Jon Watkins, the happy-to-cut surgeon popped his head round the door. "How are things going, Dan?"
"Splendid!" Dan told him. "I'll be here a few minutes more though."
"Take your time, got a late notice golf game to arrange tomorrow, buddy!" Jon called as he dashed off to the coffee-machine, with his mobile phone pressed tightly to his ear.

Dan tormented the patient a little longer, and then applied a slug of Pancuronium, a long-lasting muscle relaxant.
Picking up the Propofol syringe, he said, "Tonight, I am your God. I'll decide whether or not you wake up. I'm surprised no one ever told you this before: Never, ever piss your anuesthetist off! Especially before the operation! That's just common sense. How stupid can you get?"

Metro Cop

It was six o'clock in the morning. Dr Billy Beagle, an obstetrician, was laying rubber, as he sped down the road in his new Mercedes 500SL. He had been summonsed by a mid-wife in the obstetrics unit at St Martin's hospital. A mother-of-two was progressing very slowly with her third child. She had been in active labour for a few hours, but her cervix dilation was moving at less than two centimetres an hour. This is disconcerting for women who have already experienced a normal natural birth. The mid-wife became concerned. They had reached the point where an obstetrician was required to decide whether or not an emergency caesarean should be carried out.

Mitch the Metro Cop was hiding behind a tree along a stretch of road, where the speed limit was sixty kilometres an hour. He aligned his radar gun with the road. He was just in time to zap Billy doing a hundred and twenty. Gleefully, Mitch jumped into the road and waved Billy over to the side. He swaggered slowly towards the car, practising the cowboy gait he so admired in the movies.

Billy wound down his window impatiently; hoping the dickhead-cop would just hurry along, and either give him a ticket or let him go. Mitch finally arrived at the window. "Good morning, and where were you flying to?" he asked sarcastically. In no mood to fanny about, Billy snapped, "I am a doctor with a medical emergency to attend to. Give me a ticket or let me go!"

Mitch was enjoying his position of power too much to let the moment pass so quickly. "What kind of emergency?" he asked stubbornly.

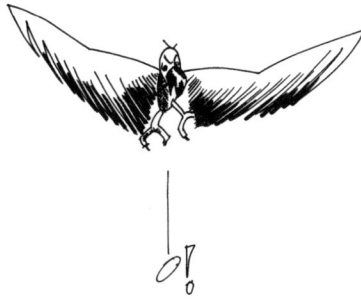

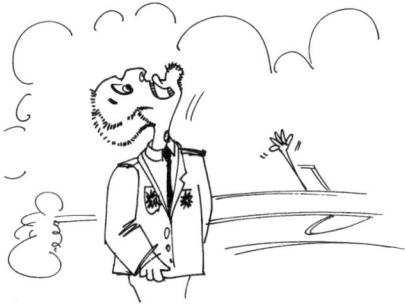

"A dire emergency – what other kind is there? I have a pregnant woman who needs an emergency caesarean and I don't have time for this crap!" Billy shouted.

"Well, you could kill someone driving at that speed!" Mitch sniffed, hitching up his belt and puffing out his chest. "Two people might die if you don't hurry up with the ticket or let me go!" Billy growled through gritted teeth.

Mitch sniffed again, and made a big production of finding the right page in his ticket pad. "I'm going to give you a ticket. It won't take long. What's your name?"

"Dr Billy Beagle."

"Dr what? Eagle? Like the bird that soars and shits in the sky?" Mitch thought he was being clever.

"No. Beagle like the dog whose shit you must have trodden in when you were behind that tree!" Billy wrinkled his nose and looked pointedly at Mitch's shiny boots. Unable to resist checking, Mitch lifted his feet one at a time. When he saw that they were clean, he glared at Billy and gave him a ticket for the maximum fine.

Defibrillator Genius

The Defence Force encourages its troops to participate in basic life support courses, to bolster its cardio pulmonary resuscitation (CPS) skills throughout the ranks. Five young lads, fresh out of school, were recruited into the medical division at the local military base and were nominated, without delay, to partake in an advanced life saving course.

Here they learnt about the defibrillator; a very handy piece of medical equipment to have around when the fear of being shot is almost constant. An expert explained how it worked, where to place the paddles or pads, and how to use the power settings.

The eager recruits nodded sagely as they learnt that patients should ideally be unconscious, before they received several volts to the heart. You'd think it was obvious.

The tutor left that evening, leaving instructions for the men to familiarise themselves with the training manual and emergency equipment. It was a lot to take on board, and their heads were spinning with the new information.

One of the recruits, Olly, was not what one would call a rocket scientist. He hadn't bothered to finish school, and was ineligible for admission to any university. In fact, his options were limited to flipping burgers in McDonalds, or joining the army. He decided that the army was his best bet. The uniform was cool, he'd get to play with guns, and he wouldn't have to be nice to people all day.

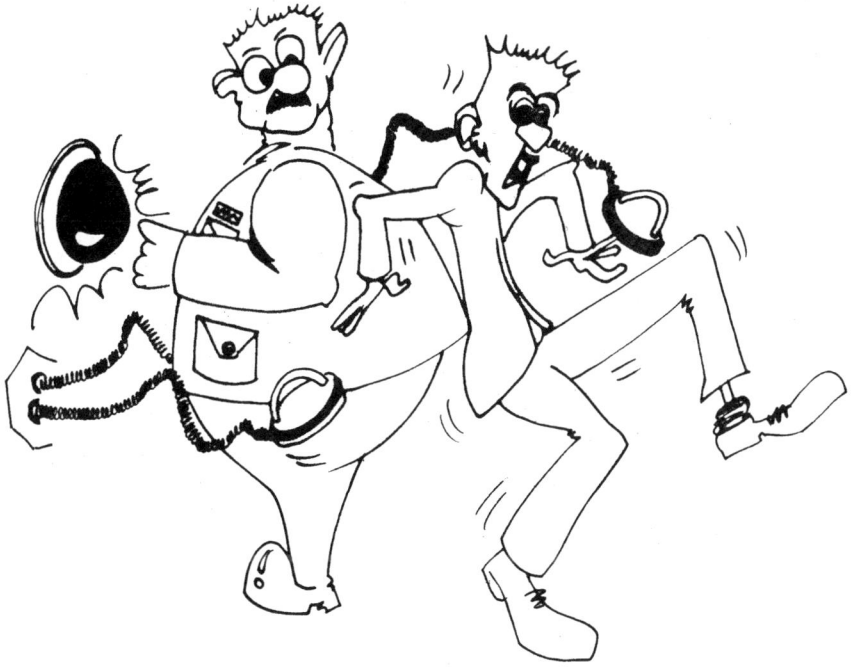

He decided to show the others how the defibrillator thing was done. He grabbed the paddles, placed one on the front of his thigh, and the other on the inside of his knee. Had he checked, he would have noticed that the power setting was at 200J.

Watched nervously by his mates, Olly pressed the red buttons. Everyone heard the loud "snap," and saw the flash of bright light. Olly let out a loud wail, and fell to the floor as the smell of singed bacon assailed the nostrils of the onlookers.

His stupidity left him with third degree burns, a fractured femur, and long-term rehabilitation ahead. The damage to his ego hurt more than his continuing limp. We should all sleep well at night, knowing that our lives are in such competent hands, wouldn't you say?

Manic Confusion

Depression and mania are common symptoms of Bipolar Disorder. The moods can range from a general feeling of being down-in-the-dumps, to the sufferer experiencing uncontrolled psychotic outbursts. Bipolar depressives have symptoms of major depression and mania: an elevated state of wellness, activity and invincibility. Patients who slip into a psychotic manic episode, may also become extremely physically powerful, and very difficult to rationalise with. Those who continually slip into mania, may be treated with long-term doses of lithium. Those who omit to take their dose of lithium, in the mistaken belief that they are cured, could find themselves slipping into such uncontrolled states of mania.

2 a.m.

It was Sunday morning, the twenty-ninth of March. Payday. I sat working myself to death, surrounded by psychos, alcoholics, Munchausen specials, criminals and a small minority of normal, decent sick people. I was getting tired of loud drunk people dripping blood on my desk, my medical notes, and the floor around me. Should I be feeling like this, only a year after qualifying as a casualty doctor? My family and friends would be sleeping. I could only yearn for my comfortable bed.

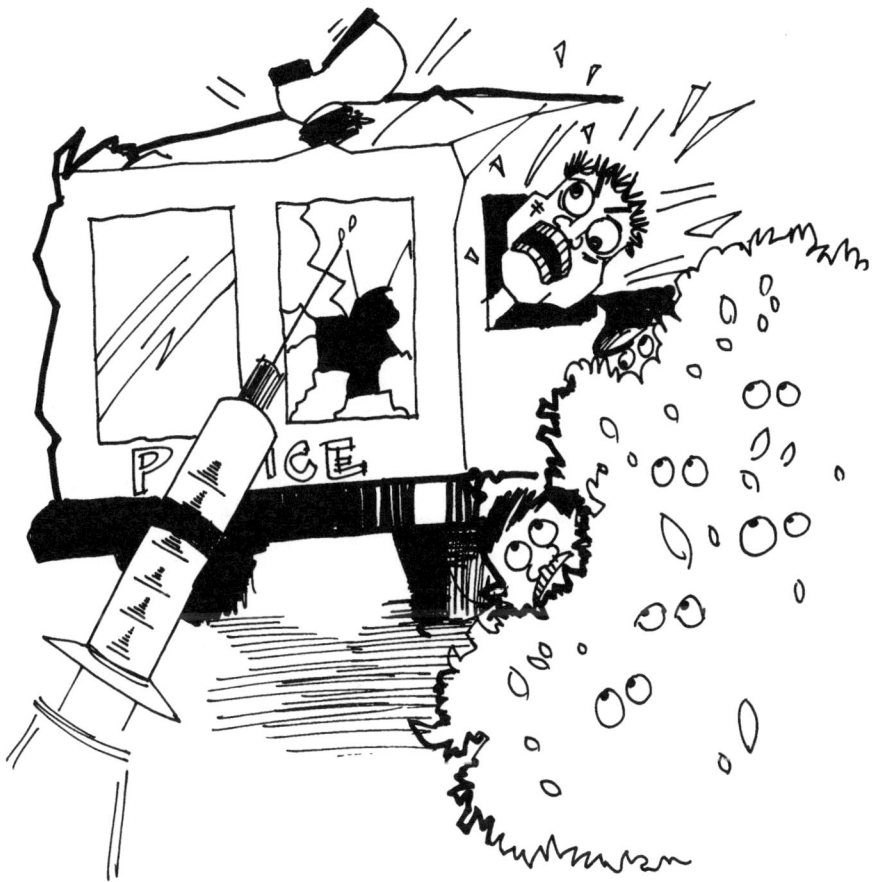

Paydays were always the same. Many poor people would take what little they had, spending it on possibly the worst drug in the world – alcohol. These pathetic creatures would create an artificial joyful state for themselves; that would last only a few short hours, before they were brought crashing back to earth by a violent criminal intervention, involving assault and theft of what little they had at the time.

The paddlers call this phenomenon a hydraulic. I prefer to look at it as an urban vicious futile circle.

3 a.m.

A pale policeman scrambled in. "Doc, we need your help, now!"

I followed him outside to a yellow police truck, surrounded by five armed policemen, parked in the ambulance zone. Intermittently, loud banging erupted inside the truck. The vehicle shuddered and rocked, as if in a violent rage. It sounded as if there was a prehistoric predator locked up in the back, setting a similar scene to the blockbuster, Jurassic Park. It gave me the chills.

"Doc, we need you to go in and sedate this mad patient!" a policeman told me, his eyes bulging with fright. I was quite sure this kind of work was not in my job description. We could see the metal sides of the truck bulge with each forceful bang that came from inside, causing flakes of yellow paint to fall off on the outside.

I stared at the cops in amazement. "You want me to go in there alone, with a syringe and needle, while six cops wait outside?" The cops nodded, eagerly. "Are you stark staring mad?" I shouted. "Who's in there anyway?"

"Don't worry, Doc, it's only big Lucian Cook; the bipolar depressive. He's actually ok until he becomes manic!" The cop did his best but I was not convinced. "He probably forgot to take his medication again."

I began to shake. "So I'm expected to go in there, with a syringe full of etamine, and persuade him to relinquish himself to me so that I can give him a sleeping injection?" The cops shook their heads.

"No Doc, you can't talk to him – he's too crazy for that! You'll have to run at him, and quickly stab him in the arm. Make sure he doesn't get hold of you though, or he'll throw you around in there!"

"I'm a doctor not a safari vet! This isn't the Serengeti, and I don't have a tranquilliser gun!" I protested. "Listen, there are seven of us. Let's use our combined strength to restrain him, and then I can sedate him." I thought this a very clever plan. I certainly was not going in there alone.

We arranged for two security guards and four porters to assist us with the task of getting the patient onto the floor long enough for me to deliver a sedating shot.

4 a.m.

Twelve men and I stood behind the police truck. I aspirated twenty millimetres of etamine out of the glass vial. A nurse placed cushions on the ground, to reduce the chance of injury to the patient as we pulled him out. The plan was to open the door, coaxing the patient out as gently as possible, then position him in such a way that I could jab him. Actually, it sounded just like a game capture!

"Are we all ok with the plan, men?" I checked with the troops. They claimed that they were ready for action. I was scared to death but couldn't show it.

4.30 a.m.

The bolt was pulled back and the back door of the truck unlocked. Silence. We waited.

4.40 a.m.

Suddenly the door was flung open and chaos erupted. Big Lucian threw himself onto the twelve men standing outside in a bizarre stage-dive. The men collapsed under his weight. Screams and groans came from the writhing mass of bodies. I sweated with fear. I darted in to select the appropriate buttocks into which I could administer my drug. I stabbed, injected and withdrew.

4.45 a.m.

The mass began to disperse. To my horror, Lucian jumped up, using four bodies to balance himself. He head-butted a policeman, and broke into a fast gallop across the parking lot, disappearing quickly into the darkness of the night.

4.50 a.m.

I was amazed! 20mls of Etamine is enough to drop anyone.

The remaining policemen and guards arose, battered and bruised. The porters received the brunt of the maniac's rage. Soon everyone was back on his feet – except Bernie, who lay semi-comatose.

I quickly checked him over for injuries, and found nothing but a bloodstain on his buttock. Oops!

5 a.m.

We carried Bernie inside, and put him on a trolley for the rest of the night. The police began to search the town for the escaped maniac. The porters refused to get involved in such dangerous activities, and the security guards dismissed themselves three hours earlier than usual.

9 a.m.

Guilt-ridden, I wrote Bernie a note of apology, which he would be able to read when he woke up - in about eight hours! I went home.

Doctor Warden

Jack's 'compulsory medical service year' began when the State placed him in a densely populated third world homeland area. He had to provide the usual clinic and surgery services, as well as fulfilling his prison and morgue duties, if he wanted to get his complete medical certification that is.

Dressed in his white coat with a stethoscope hanging around his neck, Jack was picked up by two prison wardens, Sipho and Thomas. They were to transport him to the prison, where he would begin his first day of work.

Along the way, Thomas announced that they had to make a quick stop to pick up a prisoner. Jack nodded absently. When they arrived at the police station, Sipho reached behind his seat, pulling out a Kalashnikov semi-automatic rifle. Noticing Jack's raised eyebrows, Thomas took great delight in explaining that the prisoner they were collecting had been jailed for armed robbery, and was considered extremely dangerous.

Jack swallowed a lump of fear: their mode of transport was a pick-up truck, and he couldn't help wondering where the prisoner was going to sit. His relief was evident when, a short while later, they drove off with Sipho and the prisoner, hands cuffed to feet, in the

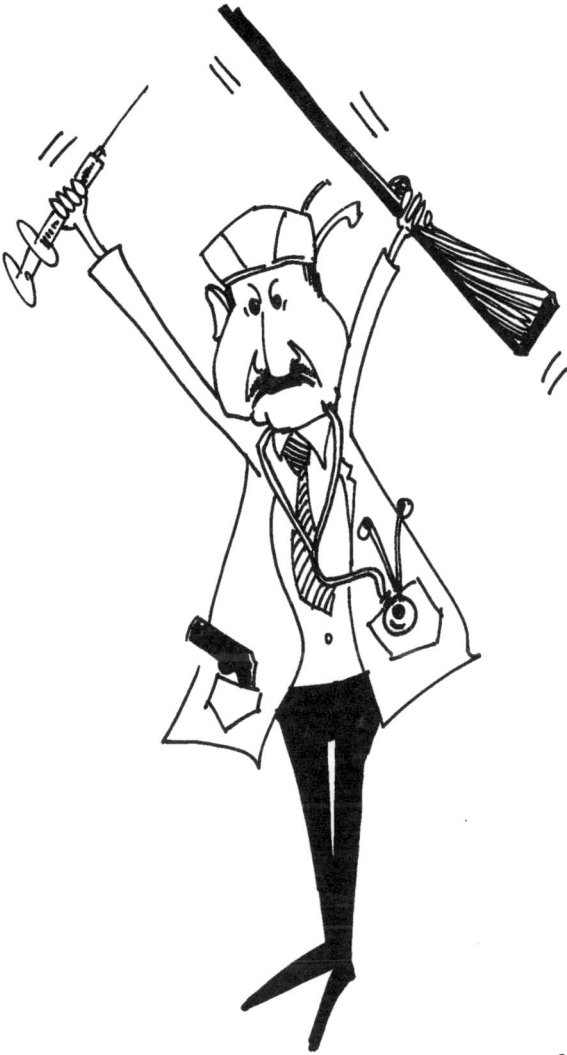

— TO GIVE OR TAKE AWAY —

back of the pick-up. Jack's eyes kept flicking to the rear view mirror, nervously sizing up their dangerous cargo. The prisoner was a portrait of bulging muscle, covered in grotesque tattoos, no less menacing for the handcuffs, which looked flimsy against such obvious strength.

Suddenly, Thomas stopped in front of a small shop and hopped out of the cab. "Out!" he called to Jack.

Jack obeyed. "What now?" he asked, as Thomas ran around to join him.

"We have to pick up some stuff for the prison kitchen. If they don't get lunch on time, we'll have a riot on our hands. Swap places with Sipho, and cover the prisoner while we get the tins."

Before Jack could formulate an answer, Sipho had hopped off the back of the truck, handing Jack the weapon. "If he moves – shoot!" he nodded at the prisoner. The prisoner seemed to find Jack's predicament amusing. He grinned widely, showing numerous gaps in his teeth. The grin wasn't friendly. Jack was well aware that the rifle was waving around in his nervous grip.

Thomas and Sipho were back in less than five minutes. It had been long enough for Jack to realise, that when he had taken the Hippocratic Oath that bound him to preserve life, he had never once considered that he might one day find himself in a position where he may be forced to take a life.

First Consultation

Josh and Peter met at medical school. Their friendship strengthened throughout their clinic years, through good times and bad. They were lucky enough to practise their houseman and senior medical officer years together, at the same district hospital. They were both extroverts, and their senses of humour and charisma ensured that they were the life and soul of the many parties they attended.

Their friendship continued even after they met their 'special ladies.' Josh went on to marry, and undertook an Obstetric and Gynaecology postgraduate position away from the district hospital. Peter went on to locum as a General Practitioner locally, and internationally, in National Health Care hospitals. The time flew past. Five years later, Peter found himself back in the same district hospital that he had started out in. Josh completed his postgraduate degree in the government sector, and decided to purchase a specialist practice in the same rural town.

Josh had maintained contact with one of his senior fellows, with whom he had developed a good relationship a few years prior to beginning his postgraduate training rotation. They became partners. Soon Josh would be in private practice. Peter made it his business to find out exactly when Josh would begin.

During his time as a locum, Peter met many people, doctors and patients, of different cultures and ethnic backgrounds. One such person was Dr Mohammed Al-Kerrie, a Muslim practising GP. Peter and Mo were very tolerant of each other's cultures, and spent hours in good-natured debates on a variety of issues. Peter had a very

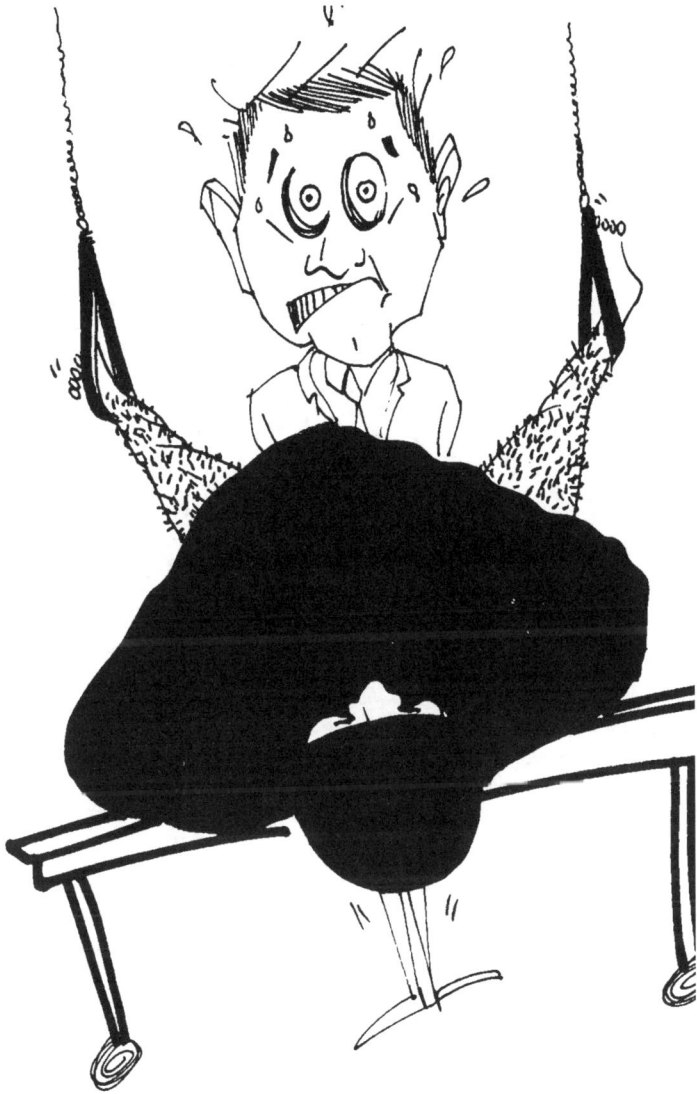

persuasive nature, and so it came about that Mo agreed to take part in a practical joke that had the potential to be hilarious.

Peter told Mo that he had spoken to Josh's secretary, and registered as Josh's first consultation. Peter smirked as he outlined his plan. Mo went off to his cousin, Kishore, and borrowed a Chandor

Chari and Hijab – the garments worn by Muslim women.

At ten-thirty on Thursday morning, Mr Al-Alsan entered Josh's surgery. He was accompanied by his submissive wife; dressed from head to toe in the traditional black robe and veil. Mrs Al-Alsan obediently followed her husband into the consulting room, where they were greeted by Josh. Mr Al-Alsan, in heavily accented English, managed to explain that it was customary for him to speak on behalf of his wife, and that Josh should direct all his questions to him. He would then translate such questions into Arabic, so that his wife would understand. Of course, this did nothing to put Josh at ease on his first consultation.

"So what appears to be the problem?" he asked Mr Al-Alsan.
"I have recently been married to my wife, who travelled here all the way from Iran. My parents introduced her to me. We have a little problem." Josh waited to see if Mr Al-Alsan would be a bit more specific. Mr Al-Alsan spoke boldly to his wife and she whispered something in his ear. It seemed she suffered from dyspareunia – a condition characterised by pain during sexual intercourse. "It also hurts me when I…" Mr Al-Alsan finished his sentence with a shrug and sheepish nod of his head.

Josh began to take a detailed account of Mrs Al-Alsan's history, covering everything from local vaginal infections and cycle abnormalities, to psychological aetiologies and drug history. The information he was given left him with no idea what the problem could be. Whenever he asked a question, the patients were vague, delivering an inappropriate explanation. Josh was finding the three-way communication method quite off-putting, and was becoming more confused as the consultation progressed. He was also under pressure, as it was his first consultation and he didn't want to disappoint his new partner.

"I'll need to examine your wife in the treatment room," he eventually told Mr Al-Alsan. "Please ask her to lie down on the examination table, and wait for me. I'll be putting her in an uncomfortable position, so that I can examine her internally using a speculum. This device will allow me to look for the cause of the problem. I will also take a pap smear from the mouth of the cervix." Mr Al-Alsan addressed his wife, and she answered with a half-bow.

In the treatment room, Josh asked her to put her feet into the stirrups, which she proceeded to do, after her husband translated from the other side of the curtain. Josh couldn't help but notice the bushy deposits of hair on Mrs Al-Alsan's feet. He slowly rolled the black robe back over her knees, finding that the hair on her legs was denser than that on her feet. As her pelvic area came into view, Josh shuddered. Never in his gynaecological career had he seen such a sight. Between the bulky thighs, tufts of thick black hair and folds of skin, lay a root-like organ, peering out at him. It was like a Cabonossi sausage, dropped down towards the perineal area.

Josh jumped back, quickly whipping the robe back into place. He cleared his throat several times before attempting to speak to Mr Al-Alsan. "Mr Al-Alsan...I can now see what is causing your wife's discomfort. I...er...did your parents check the ...er...Iranian merchandise before it left the port?"
Mr Al-Alsan lowered his brows. "What do you mean?" he growled.

Josh became very nervous. He was aware that he might ignite a huge dispute right there in his office, on his first day; and in hearing range of ten ladies who were waiting in reception. He needed to choose his words very carefully. "The pain you two experience is due to her...bum – his bum..."

"Whaat?" Mr Al-Alsan didn't seem to like what Josh was alluding to. "What do you mean?" he shouted.
As Josh paled the robed figure began to shake. A wicked laugh came through the veil. As Mo joined Peter in laughing hysterically, Josh managed a pale grin of relief.

Erection of the Dead

The dissection year of med-school is a journey into the anatomical world of the human body. Each student has an ethical responsibility to treat his assigned corpse with the utmost respect. Unfortunately, there are always a couple of jokers who ignore the rules.

Jon the Joker was a straight-A student. He was also misguided and mischievous. The other students in his class suspected that he had the hots for Jessica Stevens, but he would never admit it. Jessica looked like a cloned version of Kate Moss: fine ass; bad attitude; regal gait and a gold card. She was also terrified of cadavers – something of a problem in a dissection hall – and could be spotted a mile off, wearing enough quarantine gear to make you think there was an Ebola scare.

This particular afternoon, Jon got to the dissection hall early, with mischief in mind. He worked swiftly on a cadaver, channelling a superficial plane under the skin (tough and rigid due to the formalin and rigor mortis processes) between the collarbone and the base of the penis. When this was done, he ran a fishing line through the plane, and connected it to the larger-than-average penis. He connected the other end to a stirrup, which hung under the table.

Jessica strutted into the hall, wearing a designer floral dress, which she would swap for her hazard suit before class started. Jon and three other students surrounded the table. "Jessica?" Jon beckoned her over.

She walked slowly to the table. Jon's friends watched in anticipation. "What do you naughty boys want?" Jessica lisped as she approached the feet-end of the table.

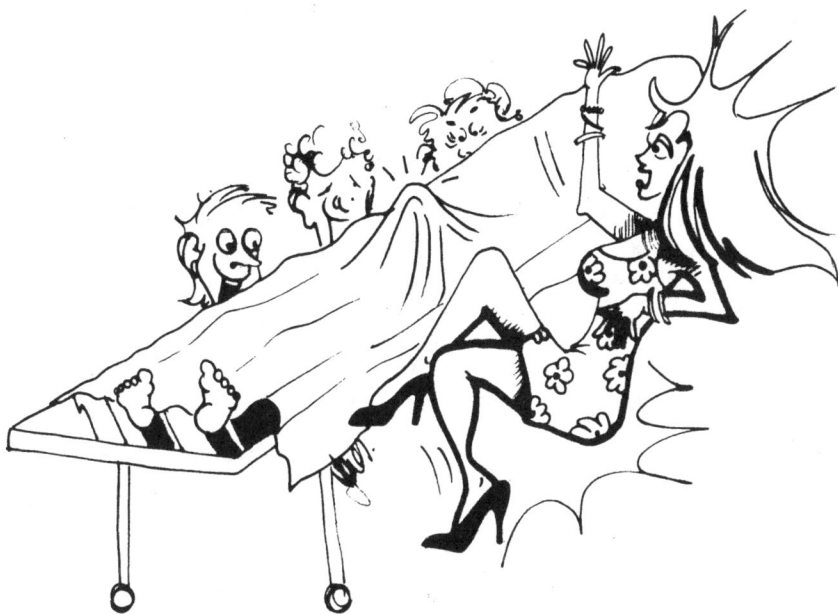

Jon used his foot to coax the stirrup down, and the cadaver's penis began to rise right before Jessica's horrified eyes. As she screamed, she threw herself backwards to get away from the moving corpse, and was rewarded with a bruised coccyx and a massive dent to her ego, as the other students howled with laughter.

Dining on a Dodgy Digit

Dudley, a continental waiter, had been employed at the fabulous Oak Plantation Restaurant for many years. As he came with excellent references, management had had no qualms about hiring him. He had given them no reason to regret their decision. So, when regular customers such as the Jacobs family arrived to celebrate Sarah's fifth birthday, Dudley was tasked with ensuring that they receive service of the highest quality.

No one noticed the wince of pain that flitted across Dudley's face, as he stood with his hands behind his back, reciting the specials of the day. Orders were placed, and the party of seven settled down to enjoy their drinks, catching up on each other's news.

The first course arrived. Rob Jacobs experienced a moment of unease when Dudley placed a bowl of Lemongrass soup in front of him. There was nothing wrong with the soup, but Rob couldn't help but notice that Dudley's thumb was fully submerged in the usually delicious broth. Not wanting to make a fuss at a happy family occasion, Rob accepted Dudley's enthusiastic encouragement to enjoy his food, but remained unimpressed when Dudley strolled away, sucking his thumb.

As the drinks and conversation flowed, Rob managed to push the incident to the back of his mind. That is, until the main course arrived.

A great one for forward planning, Liz Jacobs had decided at the time of the booking a week earlier, that she would have the Shepherd's Pie, a perfectly spiced mince meat with a hint of mint,

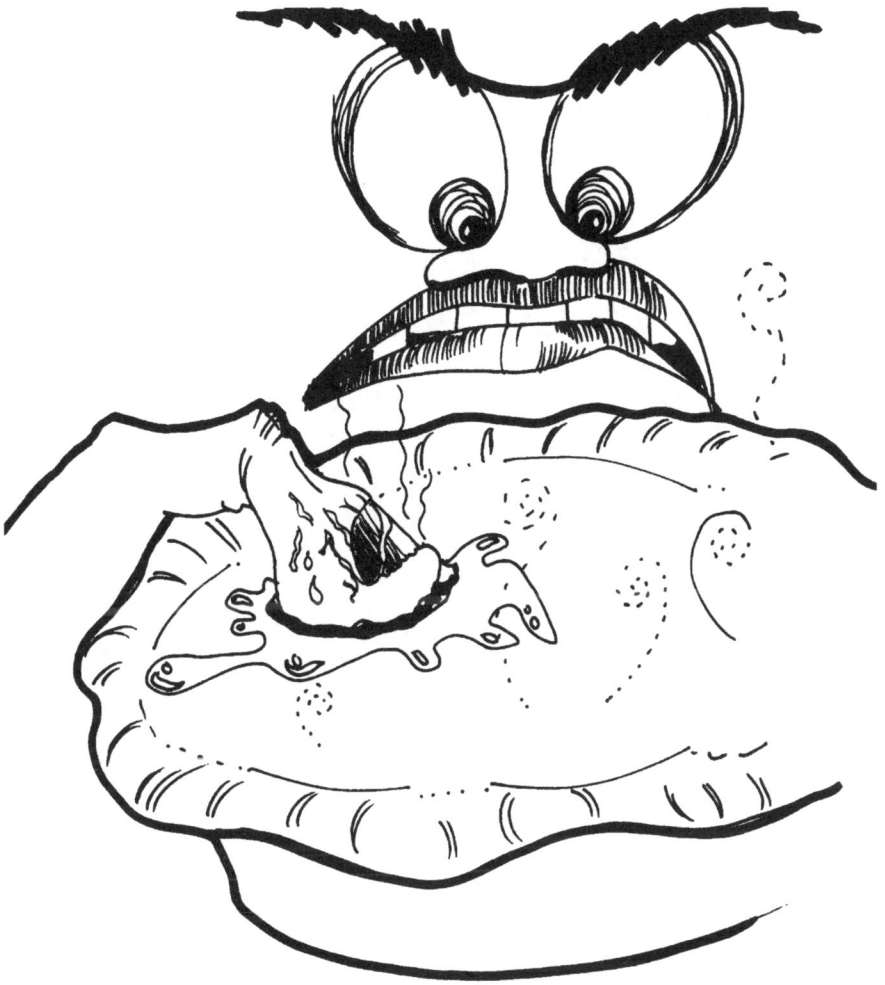

topped with a golden crust. Her taste buds retreated in disgust, as she noticed Dudley's thumb buried deep into the crust, causing thick gravy to bubble up from the indentation when the thumb was removed. She cast a quick glance at Rob who grimaced and shrugged as if to say, "Go ahead and make a fuss if you want to!"

But Liz didn't like to cause trouble. Also, Dudley was being so sweet to little Sarah as he presented her with a plate of sausage and chips, that she decided to overlook his trespass into her pie. Her patience was sorely tried, however, when Dudley stuck his thumb in his mouth as he sauntered back to the kitchen.

Two things puzzled Rob. Firstly, how did Dudley stand the heat of the food brought fresh from the kitchen? Secondly, he didn't seem at all apologetic about thumbing their food. Rob craned his neck to see if there were signs of thumbing going on at the other tables Dudley was serving, but all seemed to be in order. He then watched Lynton's face for any sign of amusement, since he was known for his practical jokes, and could easily have set the whole thing up. Again, nothing seemed out of the ordinary.

The wining and dining continued. Dudley was all smiles, checking that everyone was enjoying the meal. Matters came to a head, when Lynton's pan-fried crepes were served ... complete with Dudley's thumb jammed into one end. Lynton didn't have much truck with diplomacy, and didn't take kindly to having his favourite dessert tampered with.

"What the hell are you doing sticking your thumb in my crack?" he roared, leaping up from his chair, and causing great consternation among the other diners. Especially those who didn't have the advantage of seeing which crack Lynton was referring to.

Dudley stood shame-faced, blackcurrant sauce dripping from his thumb. He reached into his jacket, and pulled out a leaflet he'd picked up at the doctor's surgery. Rob and Lynton snatched the leaflet away, and skimmed over a couple of paragraphs about using ice packs to reduce inflammation after certain injuries. As Dudley stuck his thumb in his mouth, they read with growing alarm the section that recommended heat packs for similar injuries.

They both looked at Dudley in disbelief, as he removed his thumb from his mouth, and showed them the offending digit. It was red and swollen like a lollipop, oozing, with bits of skin flaking off around the edge. Dudley sobbed that the warm food had been his only remedy for the pain over the last four days.

Screeching with horror, Liz stood up and tried to handbag him, as management raced to the scene. As the angry mob chased him through a side door, Dudley thanked his lucky stars that his feet weren't similarly afflicted.

Dudley and his abscess have since been notably absent from the Oak Plantation Restaurant.

Stupid Surgeon

Surgeons are a unique group of people, all aiming for the same ultimate clinical goal, with varying degrees of success. The general consensus of hospital staff is that surgeons are temperamental. This could mean mild mannered one minute, and short tempered the next; histrionic then calm; easy-going then pedantic. Or, if you want to call a scalpel a scalpel, "belligerent bastards" may be the description we are looking for.

A surgeon can appear rational and sympathetic when conversing with a patient, offering a comforting confidence that convinces patients that they are in good hands. But, once the patient is unconscious and stretched out on the operating table, the same surgeon can exhibit signs of borderline multi-personality disorder. The last thing you would expect is for a surgeon to have a stampy-feet, hissy fit as he wields the scalpel.

Max, a vascular surgeon, is an intelligent, outgoing chap, with a beautiful wife and adoring kids. He enjoys a few beers as much as the next man, and always makes time to walk his dog. His bedside manner during clinical consultations can't be faulted: An all round good bloke.

Until he gets into theatre. Then the surgical greens he pulls on may as well be a devil's costume; complete with horns, pointy tail and scalpel in place of a trident. The nursing staff bear the brunt of his caustic tongue, tolerating the screamed curses and abusive remarks, dodging the surgical instruments and other apparatus that Max throws to any one of the four corners of his theatre.

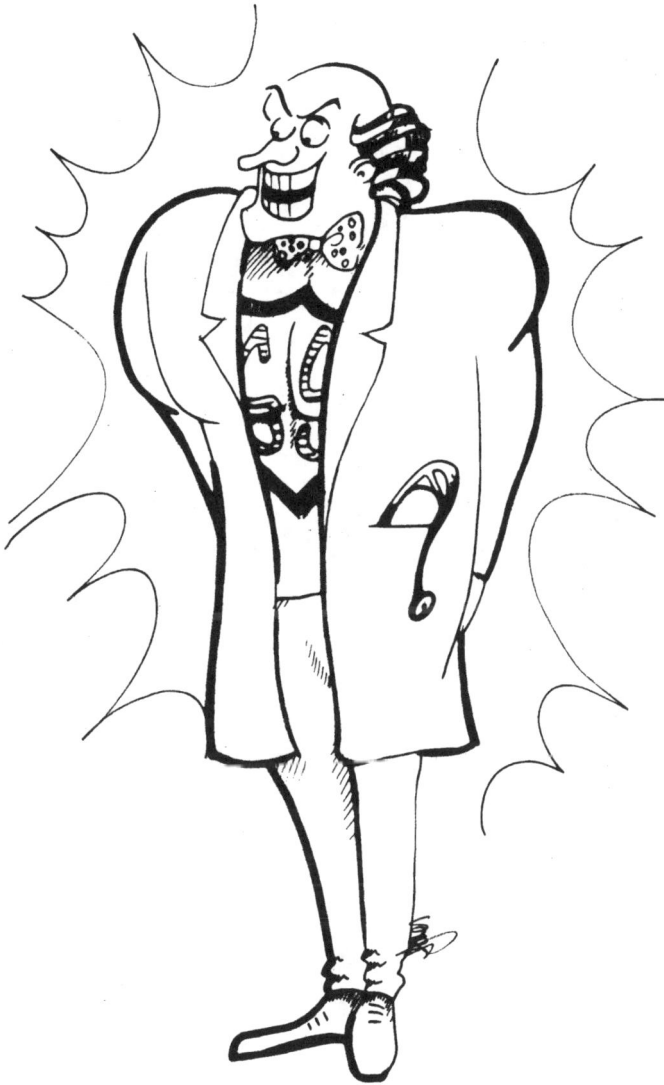

Whilst trusting patients regard their surgeons as superheroes, there are many hospital staff who would love to see such badly behaved individuals taught a stern lesson. To be given pause for thought, and reason to reflect on their outrageous behaviour.

Max's Day of Reckoning came quite unexpectedly. Those who witnessed his downfall had Mr. Watson to thank for it.

Mr. Watson had a hernia and was relying on Max to fix him up. Since he also had a respiratory disorder, the risks of having a general anaesthetic were deemed too high. He was given a local spinal block instead. He was wheeled into theatre fully conscious, numb from the belly button down. His expression betrayed his anxious state, as he lay quietly awaiting his operation. Not that he'd have been able to dance around to kill time, even if he'd wanted to. He kept reminding himself that Max had carried out countless operations, and hadn't lost one yet. Not that operating on a hernia is considered a particularly high risk, but then no one is relaxed while waiting to go under the knife.

It was probably just as well that Mr Watson didn't know that Max would not, in fact, be performing the operation. He had handed the job over to Andrew, the registrar or Specialist in Training. This is common practice in academic institutions. The registrar will carry out certain operations, depending on his or her experience. The consultant will perform the more complicated procedures, assisted by the registrar. Occasionally, a consultant might sneak into theatre, to see how the registrar was doing during an operation.

Once the scrub sister had cleaned the area around the conscious Mr. Watson's groin, and covered him from head to toe in green sterile drapes, Andrew could begin. The operation was proceeding nicely. The anaesthetist would occasionally ask, "How are you feeling Mr. Watson?" to which the tremulous reply would filter through the drapes, "Just fine, I think."

Andrew was concentrating hard on Mr. Watson's groin, failing to notice Max slip quietly into the theatre. He snuck right up behind Andrew, before roaring "What the hell are you doing? It looks like a f***ing dog's breakfast!"

The fright caused Andrew to jump forward as if he'd been nudged with an electric cattle prod, dropping his scalpel and ending up sprawled over Mr. Watson's groin area.

Before Andrew had a chance to gather his wits, the drapes seemed to come alive, rising like a green slime monster. Mr. Watson sat bolt upright, demanding to know what the hell was going on, as he fought to find a way out from under the drapes. Shell-shocked, Andrew slid to the floor with a thud, coming to rest somewhere between the suction unit and the swab counting rack. A nurse rushed to his side, more to be out of the line of fire, than out of concern for poor Andrew.

Max had stood frozen to the spot for the few seconds that it took for the results of his rash behaviour to unfold. His face took on a sickly hue when he realised that the patient wasn't under general anaesthetic, but was instead fully conscious and aware that Max had caused mayhem with his ill-judged outburst.

He racked his brain trying to come up with a way to blame someone else for the horrifying scene before him. Andrew was being helped to his feet, dazed and shocked. The anaesthetist was trying to placate Mr. Watson, who didn't know whether he was terrified or furious, attempting to have both emotions at the same time. Max knew he couldn't wriggle out of this one. Muttering a subdued sorry, he turned and departed from the theatre with as much dignity as he could muster.

It took four times the normal sedation dose to calm Mr. Watson. He needed to be convinced that the operation had to be completed, because walking around with a gaping hole in his groin would not be in his best interests.

Although Max is now much better behaved in theatre, he has trouble sleeping. But that's hardly surprising, given the medico-legal investigation that is pending.

Oklahoma Bomber

In July 2002, a colleague of mine was making the most of a quiet moment in the theatre complex. Goose sat with his feet up and the newspaper spread across his legs, scanning for snippets of interesting news. An article about the death sentence handed down to the Oklahoma bomber caught his eye. The convicted man was due to die by lethal injection. It was the recipe and dosage of the drugs that really made Goose sit up and take notice. He read the article carefully. When he had finished a humorous grin spread across his face.

A couple of years before, Goose had worked at a two-hundred-bed African bush hospital, where he was one of five doctors serving a population of twenty thousand. One day, he was in the operating room to assist with a caesarean section. He had given the obese patient a spinal anaesthesia. The obstetrician had just begun the procedure, when Goose was called to help an unconscious patient in the accident and emergency ward. The shortage of staff gave Goose no choice, but to leave his awake, pregnant patient in the safe hands of the obstetrician, scrub nurse and running nurse.

"Hold the fort, Margot!" he instructed the running nurse, as he gave his patient a final check before rushing off to help with the emergency. Not five minutes later, the scrub nurse came running, calling Goose back to an unconscious patient in the operating room.

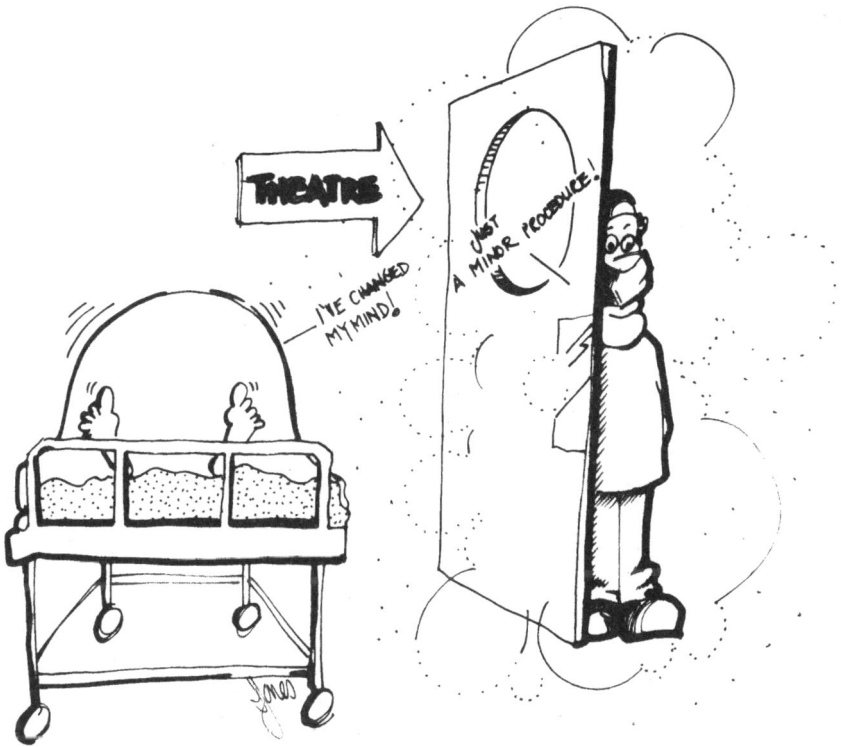

Dashing in, he found his patient was no longer breathing. Her heart rhythm had arrested. Thankfully, the baby had already been delivered.

Intubation, oxygenation and CPR were started immediately. Sixty-three shocks and a smoky theatre room later, the patient began to groan. Her cardiac function was deemed adequate, and her respiratory rate improved. She was moved into a dark quiet room to recover from her ordeal. Goose investigated what had gone wrong less than five minutes after he had rushed to the accident ward.

It turned out that when the patient complained of feeling weak, the obstetrician asked the running nurse to give the patient some intravenous glucose. Unfortunately, the fifty percent glucose is stored in the same sized glass vials as Potassium Chloride (KCL). Both vials were kept on the resuscitation trolley. The runner had failed to notice the red caution flag taped over the neck of the ampoule that said: Caution! For intravenous use, 1500 mmol KCL.

As Goose put down his newspaper, he marvelled that his resilient national health patient had survived the same rapid intravenous dose of Potassium Chloride that was used to execute the Okalahoma bomber.

(The large 50ml KCL vials are not commonly packaged that way anymore!)

Shocked Sleeping

Defibrillators use an electronic current in short bursts, to help re-synchronise an abnormal heartbeat, or in drastic cases, to restart a failed heart. The machine has two paddles, or pads, that are pressed onto or stuck to the chest, delivering a set amount of current jolts through the heart. Power settings range from 0 joules (J) to 360J. During cardiac arrest, the recommended setting starts at 200J, and can be increased if necessary.

It is important to note that patients are unconscious with no heart contraction when a defibrillator is used. Conscious patients should be sedated before the shock is delivered, as the process is very painful. And so to the shocking mishap...

Jon Turner, a relatively fit and healthy corporate executive, suddenly developed a deep burning chest pain, not accompanied by any shortness of breath or sweating. His concerned wife urged him to seek medical help immediately. A few hours later, Jon found himself in the busy cardiac department of a national hospital. He lay on a trolley, covered by a single sheet, and was connected to an electrocardiogram (ECG) which measured his heartbeat.

Jon spent a couple of hours trolley-bound. Sweating and anxious, he watched as the machine registered his heartbeats, until he fell asleep. Some time later, Nurse Peters entered the cardiac department and noticed with horror that Jon was lying very quietly. A bit too quietly for her liking, in fact. Her eyes flitted to the ECG and the trace line caused a shiver to run down her spine.

She gave a bellow for help, pushed the resuscitation trolley towards Jon's bed and charged the defibrillator to 200J as the cardiac team

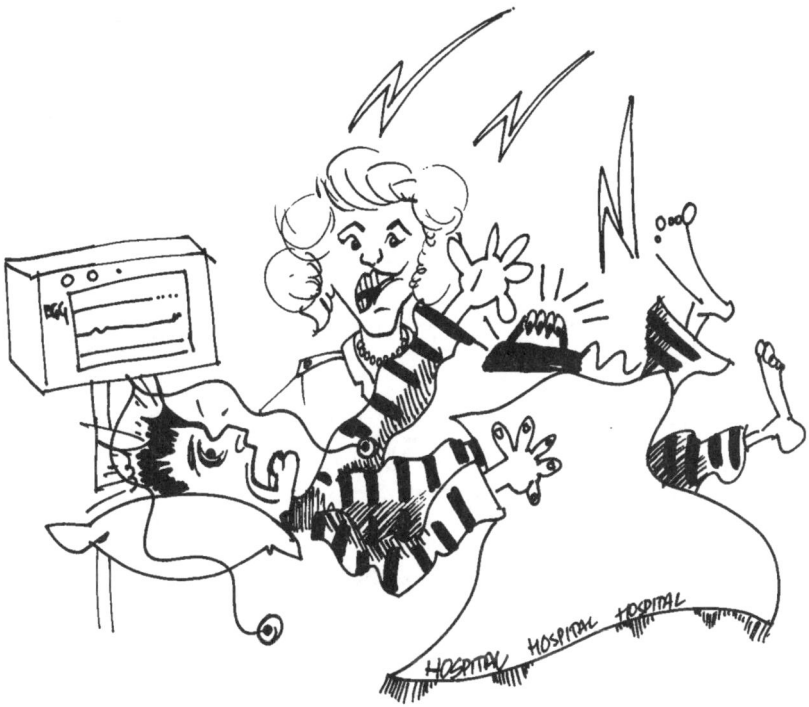

raced to her assistance. Fearing for Jon's life, Nurse Peters decided that she had to act instantly, forgetting to feel for a central pulse. She pressed the paddles to Jon's chest, and gave him a good zap.

There was a loud "thunk" as the force of the current lifted Jon's body from the bed, before dropping it seconds later. The "thunk" was immediately followed up by a shriek of pain from Jon, much to the consternation of Nurse Peters.

"What the hell are you doing? That bloody hurt!" Jon glared in indignation at the flustered Nurse. As she tried to explain herself, the cardiac team arrived and began to investigate.

It turned out that Jon's perspiration had caused the ECG stickers to fall off his chest. In her panic, Nurse Peters failed to check Jon's neck for a normal pulse. Assuming he had suffered a cardiac arrest, she had given him a good dose of electricity to wake him up. Needless to say, Jon was not impressed...

Orientation

We registered mid-January for our first year at medical school. The optimism among we 'Greens" flowed like the Nile. The schedule went as follows: registration in the morning, then an introduction in a faculty lecture auditorium. We were to be met by the senior orientation committee: ten clinical students and the Dean of Students, Dr Ron Meyers. Ron used to be Head of Department of Anatomical Pathology, and was well-known for having a good sense of humour.

The orientation committee had certain responsibilities. In spite of their own tough clinical curriculum, they had to devote time to the Greens, introducing them to the various events that occurred during the year. The first couple of days would be intense, but also offered the opportunity for a few laughs. A week prior to orientation, the committee met with Ron to discuss the initial orientation period. They decided to do something to spice up the first lecture, mocking the optimistic new medical pioneers.

New medical students are subjected to various inoculations before they are allowed to enter the microbiological realms of academic hospitals. For example, the hepatitis B virus is highly infectious and, once contracted, the prognosis is poor. Therefore, it is prudent to inoculate all students beforehand.

The auditorium is semi-circular, with thirty-five rows of seats ascending towards the back. A large white lecture table sits on the ground at the front. That afternoon, a hundred and fifty fresh-faced

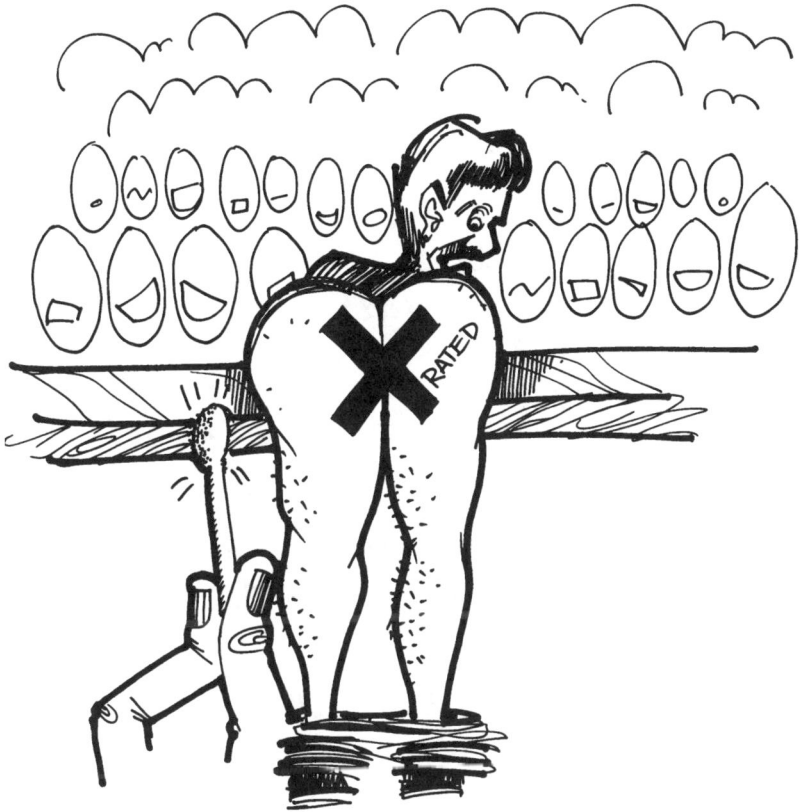

Greens sat in their civilian clothes to hear the introduction to med school. The committee, wearing white doctor-jackets, followed Ron Meyers into the auditorium, where he would give his speech.

"Ladies and gentlemen, congratulations on your acceptance into our school. You are the elite of the elite. Be aware, as you look to the person standing on either side of you, that there will be only one of them present when this year-group graduates." Satisfied that he had frightened most of the students with this statement, Ron moved on to the important business of the day: carriers of nosocomial bacteria.

"Did you know," he continued, his voice booming throughout the auditorium, "that fifteen percent of this group of students are carriers of Staphylococcus Aureus? Methelium Resistant Staphylococcus Aureus costs our National Health Service five billion pounds a year. That could buy a lot of beer!" Nervous laughter rippled through the Greens.

Ron adopted a stern expression for the next part of his speech. "This bacterium tends to grow in dark moist areas, and there is no way we are going to allow you Greens to infect our wards and intensive care patients in this institution. Hospital Health Regulation 237-3 requires us to carry out microscopy, culturing and sensitivity swab testing on each one of you. This is the only way to reduce the risk of infection in our national hospitals." Ron stuck out an arm and waved a white-coated committee member to his side. "With the help of one of your senior colleagues, we will quickly demonstrate how these procedures will work."

James Elliot bent over the white table, his rear-end pointing at Ron, and his up-turned face stared at the assembled Greens. Ron removed a twenty-centimetre swab stick from his pocket. He pulled it out of its sterile container, so the Greens could see a long thin shaft with a plastic handle at one end and a fluffy cotton bud on the swabbing end. Ron reminded them that the bacterium thrives in areas such as the armpits and anus.

Without further ado, he lifted James's white coat with his right hand, and simulated a vigorous rectal probe with his left. Ron tried not to smile as he felt the tension in the room intensify and heard uncomfortable shuffling from the front rows.

His point made, Ron stepped away from the table and James re-joined the rest of the committee.

"Ladies and gentlemen," Ron pointed at the audience, "You are the new pioneers. You are the new healthcare leaders and providers of the United Kingdom. I now need you to split up into two groups, one on each side of the auditorium, so we can get this show on the road." Ron paused to enjoy the looks of horror on the Greens' faces. "I am going to need an exceptional student, the leader of all leaders, to break the ice."

Five rows from the back, a man rose from his seat. With an arrogant smirk and swagger of confidence, he made his way down to the white table at the front. Without hesitation, he dropped his trousers and bent over the table. "To be absolutely certain of obtaining a good sample, I am going to need a three-step run-up," Ron announced as he backed up. The volunteer's smirk gave way to a look of abject fear.

Ron bounded up to the table and a loud bang echoed around the auditorium. Ron had slapped a sticky A4-sized card photo onto the Green's buttocks: a portrait of a donkey, and at the same time his knees began to buckle.

Sexual Indiscretions

People outside the medical fraternity have a continuing fascination with the sex lives of hospital personnel, and in particular, the strange and interesting locations chosen for a forbidden bonk. What better place for a passionate interlude than the sluice room? I can only imagine that such curiosity comes from watching too many hospital dramas on television. Viewers are clearly of the opinion that the bizarre and provocative relationships that exist between nurses and doctors on the screen reflect the reality in hospitals. Tight fitting white uniforms and dangling equipment, I'm talking about stethoscopes here, are giving medics a raunchy reputation they would love to deserve.

However, there was one case that could satisfy the expectations of your average armchair viewer. It involved a casualty triage nurse and a surgical trainee. Over a period of a few weeks, they had developed an intense mutual infatuation, to the point where they swapped explicit gestures and lewd suggestions even when surrounded by colleagues.

Obviously, this type of behaviour would be frowned upon by senior clinical staff and hospital management. Heaven forbid that such a professional institution should be over-run with rampant staff! I am unaware of the disciplinary procedures that would follow if a couple were caught red-handed, and undoubtedly red-faced, whilst enjoying an adult version of that old playground favourite, Doctors and Nurses!

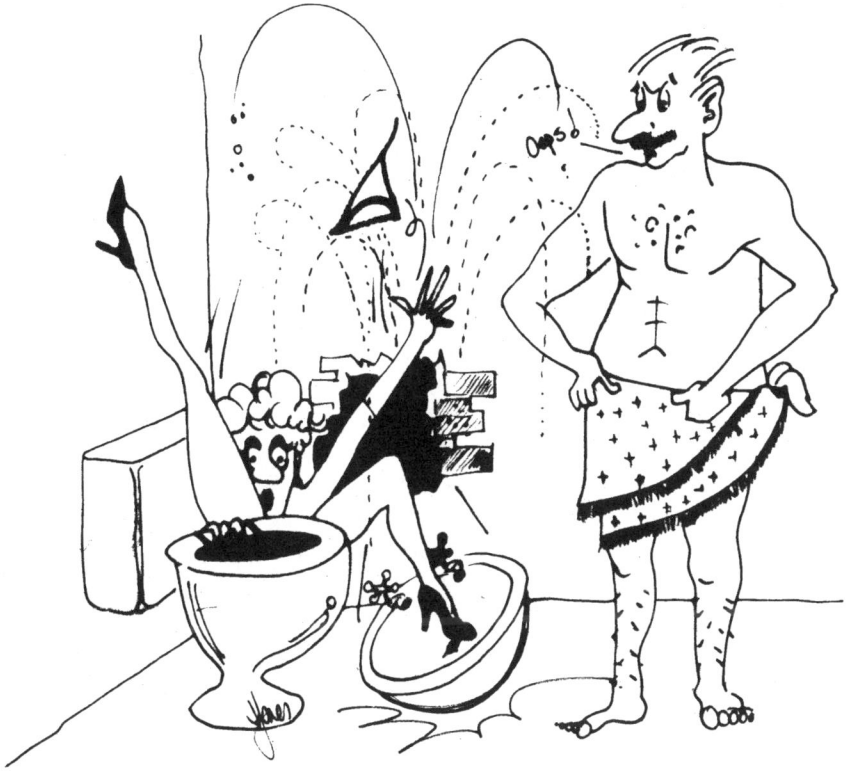

Was it something to do with working the graveyard shift? Or was it the phase of the moon? Or could it simply have been the risk of getting caught that convinced the nurse and the trainee to allow their animal instincts to prevail.

They slipped quietly into the new renal unit that was undergoing refurbishment. While most of the rooms had newly laid carpets, the bathrooms were still in a state of disrepair. Although new sinks and bathroom fittings were in place, tiles and copper piping littered the floor. Keen to avoid detection, they chose a bathroom at the farthest end of the hall, where the city lights outside provided the only illumination.

She quickly removed her underwear. He picked her up, placing her on the newly fitted sink. They kissed passionately as he loosened his belt and trousers, dropping them to the floor. Rhythmic upward thrusts were marked with gasps and groans, as they carried on with great enthusiasm.

Suddenly, at a most crucial moment, the sink plummeted to the ground with nursey still perched on top of it. The groans of ecstasy became agonised screams. To make matters worse, water gushed from the broken pipes like Niagara Falls, extinguishing their fiery passion.

To add insult to injury, the alarms then went off, bringing a trauma team storming into the flooded bathroom; only to find a highly embarrassed man, drenched and drooping, accompanied by an equally humiliated naked nurse, sporting a fractured hip, clutching a pair of knickers.

Platoon Golfer

Mike Thompson decided he needed a break from his lucrative job as an investment banker. He organised a holiday for himself, his wife and their three sons. He made reservations at a five-star hotel, which boasted a safari park, pools and a fabulous golf course. Jill would be happy to relax by the pool, while her husband took Ryan, Jon and Bruce to brush up their golfing skills. Ryan and Jon were particularly talented kids and not just on the golf course. They went to a highly regarded private school, and were leaders throughout their school careers.

Jill gave birth to Bruce after a very difficult and prolonged labour. He was eventually delivered by forceps, and had to spend many days in hospital before Mike and Jill could take him home. A few months later, he was diagnosed with Cerebral Palsy, and suffered moderate brain impairment as a result. From a young age he was subjected to intensive rehabilitation with occupational therapists doing their best to improve his speech and fine motor skills. Thankfully, he was spared the more severe symptoms of seizures, epilepsy, limb spasticity and severe mental dysfunction. After therapy, Bruce moved on to special tuition schooling at the Edington Learning Institution. When he left he found a job as a trolley porter at the General Hospital, impressing his employers with his hard work and commitment.

Bruce is a gentle guy with a good heart, but can be quite scatter-brained and impetuous. He once ran, without thinking, into a Magnetic Resonance (MR) Scan room whilst carrying an oxygen canister for a

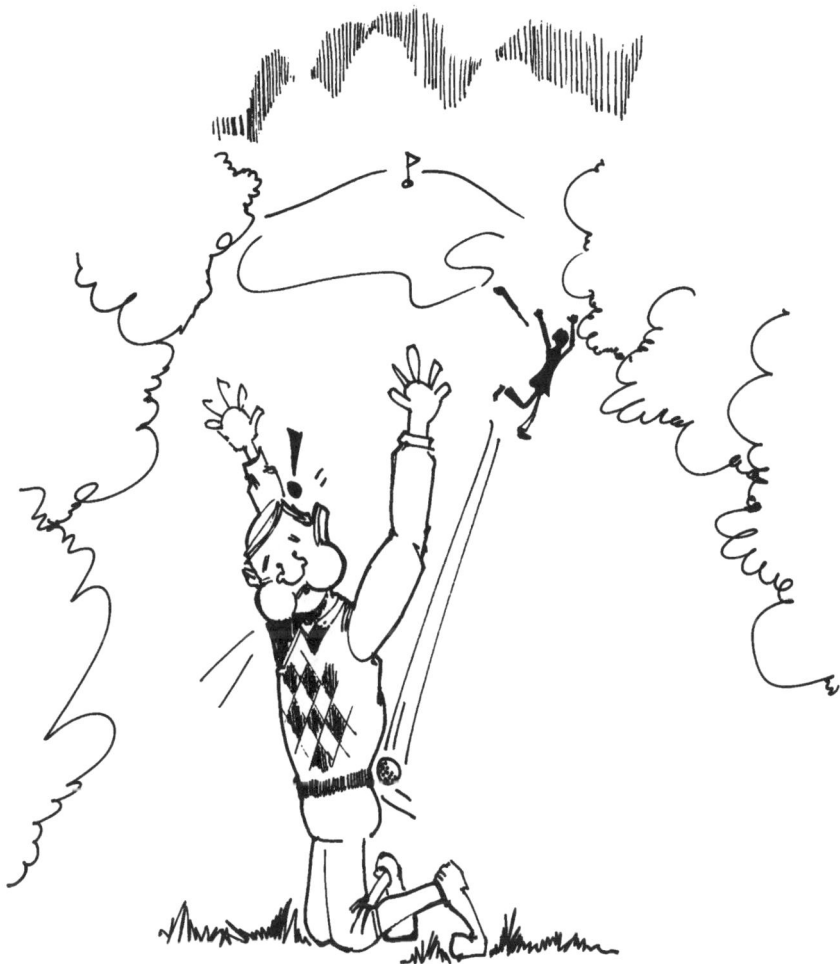

wheezy patient. It is strictly forbidden to take metal objects into the MR room. His intentions were good, but the radiology technicians were hard-pressed to say whether the clanging sound from the oxygen canister bouncing like a ping pong ball around the room was louder than the shrieks that came from the patient who was inside the scanner capsule at the time. (The lawsuit is still pending. The patient is claiming to be suffering post-traumatic stress syndrome after the terrifying event.)

On their first morning, Mike decided to take Ryan and Jon for eighteen holes of golf. Bruce demanded to join them and, since he rarely had a chance to spend time with all three of his sons together, Mike agreed. Jill took up a horizontal position on the pool deck, where she would be able to watch the men in her life tee-off.

The first tee was located in a very scenic position; just below the decking and between two palm trees; the luscious fairway bordered by tropical vegetation. Occasionally, a small animal would run across the fairway to hide in a thicket away from the golfers. Ryan, the youngest, stepped up with a wood, positioned his ball on a tee and, with a square stance, drove the ball about three hundred yards, where it landed just into the rough. Mike went next, striking the ball sweetly, so it fell short of the bunker.

The happy family scene had caught the attention of some of the guests on the patio, some of whom got up for a better view.

The Thompson men looked very professional, except for George Herman Ruth (the Babe Bruce) who was standing in the fringe of the first tee. He had become entranced by a dragonfly that was swooping through the air around him, and Bruce kept swinging his club at it. Jon had told him to stop, but Bruce took no notice. Eventually Mike yelled, "Bruce! Cut that out! It's your turn to tee-up."

Ryan positioned the ball for his brother, and Mike stood slightly in front looking down the fairway to see where the ball would land. Bruce took a Happy Gilmore run-up, and swung at the ball as hard as he could. The ball sliced off at Mach one, striking Mike square between the shoulder blades. As Mike's knees buckled, onlookers cringed as one. They were reminded of the movie, Platoon, where Willem Dafoe's character, Sgt. Elias Grodin, sinks to his knees after being shot in the back by the Viet Cong.

On his knees with his hands held high, Mike managed to groan and sob at the same time. Horrified at the pain he had inflicted upon his father, Bruce threw his club to one side, and charged back towards the hotel. He managed to side-step three guests, hurdled tables like a Thompson Gazelle, then collided with a waiter whose breakfast tray went flying through the air like a deadly metal frisbee. Bruce went into hiding, as Jill and a couple of other guests managed to lift Mike onto the back of the hotel's pick-up truck to be taken to hospital.

The Head Chef, enjoying a quick smoke-break, finally found Bruce hiding behind the kitchen bins. It took him an hour and a bottle of jellybeans to convince Bruce that his father had suffered no permanent damage, and it was safe for him to be reunited with his family.

Sangoma Magic

In African culture, curses are representative of black witchcraft. It is strongly believed that they can induce illness in an individual who believes himself to have been cursed. Therefore the first port of call in times of illness is not a western doctor, but a traditional African healer: a Sangoma.

The healing practices of Sangomas are passed down within the clans, from generation to generation and may differ according to region, tribe or village. Healing 'muti' may take the form of potions, pastes or powders made from all kinds of earthy ingredients, including berries, roots, bone pieces and dung. It is not uncommon for young patients to be admitted into hospitals suffering from complications caused by some form of traditional healing. For example, dung paste that is rubbed onto children's umbilical stumps, or detergent enemas can cause severe systemic infections, even septic shock.

Though often frowned upon by Western and scientific communities, these ancient forms of healing have been accepted by many native communities, and will be around for a few more years yet.

Tom, a new recruit, was placed in a small African bush hospital for a year. This was a major challenge, especially as there are so few doctors, so many patients and no specialist cover in the bush. Tertiary institutions can be hundreds of miles away, so the resident medical officer is left to sort out all types of medical dilemmas alone. In this situation two hands are essential: you need your left hand to

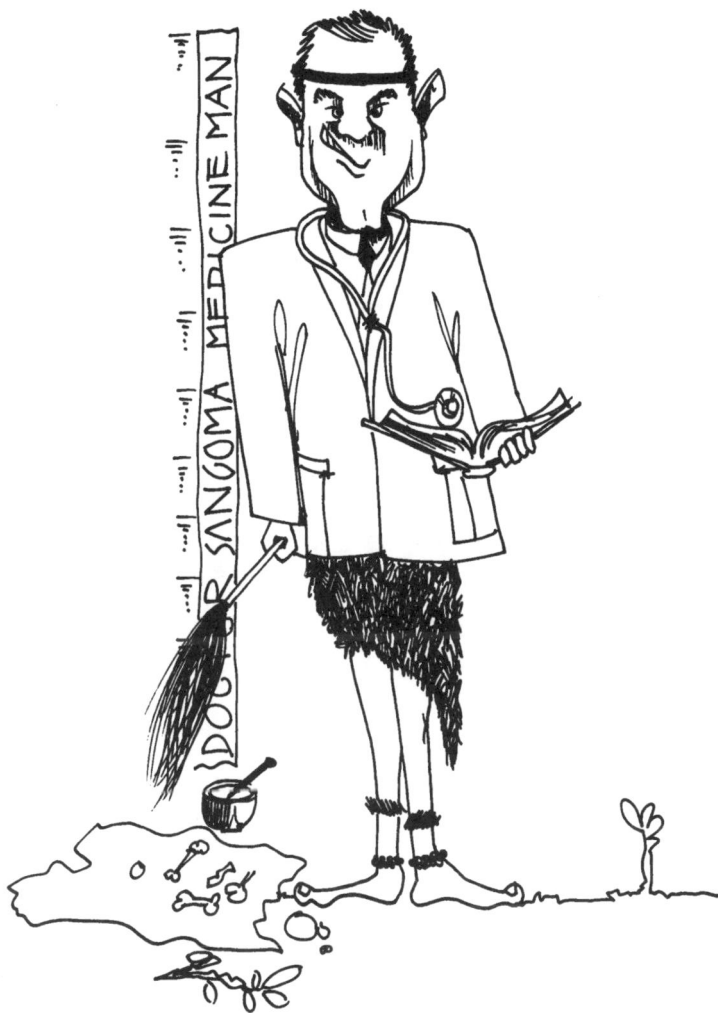

DOCTOR SANGOMA MEDICINE MAN

hold the medical book, and your right to operate. With nobody else to help you, your handbook becomes your best friend.

Tom had little orthopaedic or anaesthetic experience. In fact he had no experience whatsoever with local anaesthetic blocking techniques, which can be used where a general anaesthetic is considered too risky, for any number of reasons. Local blocking techniques are invaluable in bush hospitals because they spare patients from general anaesthesia, and help accelerate patient turn over through the operating rooms. There is the risk of complications, but statistically speaking, it is far less than those associated with general anaesthesia.

An old patient from the local tribe with a long-standing smoking history was admitted for elective orthopaedic surgery on his left hand. Tom opted to do an interscalenus block, in case the patient suffered from severe lung impairment or emphysema, which would cause complications if a general anaesthetic was used.

Of course, there was no one to show him how to do it. Tom sped through the textbook chapter describing the blocking techniques in which a local anaesthetic is applied to the nerves that run down the side of the neck to supply the arms. A specific limb, or a portion of it, can be anaesthetised for surgical intervention, while the patient is awake or asleep.

One of the uncommon side effects is an accidental block of the laryngeal nerve, which innervates the vocal cords, allowing us to talk without impairment. The block lasts for a few hours.

Tom explained what he was going to do through an interpreter nurse. The old man conversed fluently, and had no objections to this procedure, happily oblivious to Tom's lack of experience in this procedure. Positioning the patient correctly, he drew up 20mls of local anaesthetic, cleaned the neck and injected the solution. The sweat dripped from his forehead as he clenched his teeth with nervous tension.

A few minutes later the patient was still moving his left arm around every time Tom pinched him to see if it was numb. Tom became impatient, and asked him if he could feel anything. The patient had a most puzzled expression on his face and his response was, "Huuuh, nuuuh, fuuh." What the hell was going on? Tom wondered, and he quickly left the theatre to get a breather and nervously lit a cigarette.

On returning, the old man was nowhere to be found. He had discharged himself with such haste, that not even the hospital porter could catch him, as he took off through the gates in his hospital gown, ass protruding as he disappeared into the African bush.

The distressed old arthritic man legged it at surprising speed, straight to the Sangoma's hut, where a man dressed in traditional skins and bony bangles and necklaces saw him immediately. "Huuh, muuh, fuuh," he pointed desperately at his throat in a very erratic manner. The Sangoma made a swift diagnosis. After going through the motions and exchanging currency, the patient was given a bitter root to swallow and was discharged.

The old man spent the rest of the afternoon sitting on a rocky outcrop overlooking the valley, biting into the bitterest root known to the tribal people. The sweat poured out of his face, and his jawbone twitched every time he chewed. A few hours later, his voice returned at the same rate as the local anaesthetic dissipated.

Tom praised the heavens, when he happened to bump into the old patient in town, and heard him telling anyone who cared to listen about his scary escapade. A vastly relieved Tom was able to sleep better at night.

Hung like a Donkey

The late afternoon sun beat down on the Rugby Union stadium, packed to capacity. Number fourteen took five steps back and three to the side, aligning the kick in his mind. Surely he would be successful. The absolute silence in the stadium was momentarily broken by the blare of a train hooter from the nearby station. It seemed that time was standing still. Number fourteen took a slow run up, his boot hit the ball with a thud as the fans held their breath. Transfixed, they watched as the rugby ball sailed perfectly between the uprights.

The Wolves spectators came to life, rising as one, frantically cheering their team on. Only one person had no interest in the events taking place on the pitch. The occupant of Stand C, seat forty five was focussed on something entirely different. Casually, Malcolm bent down, hoping not to attract attention to himself. He checked the three litre urine catheter bag connections and strapping bound to his right inner thigh. It was three minutes to half-time. Time to put his well thought-out plan and precise anatomical craftsmanship into action. Had anyone noticed his menacing grin, they would certainly have suspected he was up to no good... and they would have been right!

The prestigious Veterinary School takes about eighty students a year. There is such a stringent selection process, that it would be absurd for a student to step out of line, or in any other way, invite disqualification. The majority of students were institutionalised. They were well aware of the political and hierarchical rules and regulations of the school, whose internal bureaucracy could match most governments. Commitment, dedication, sacrifice and a high level of academic achievement were expected from all students.

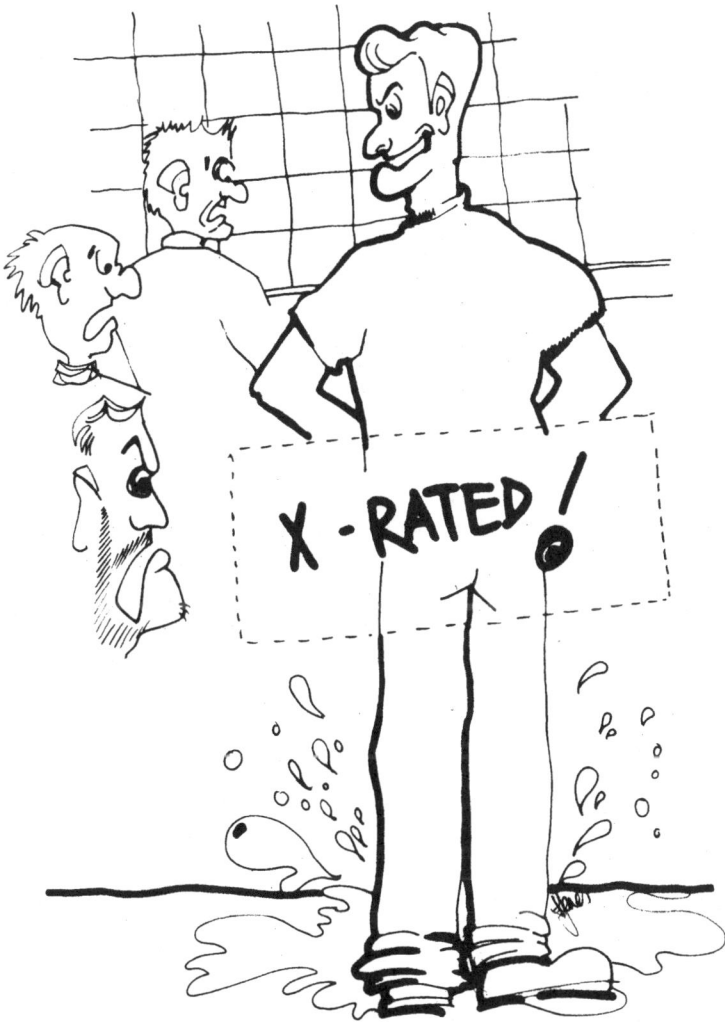

Although Malcolm's year group showed more enthusiasm, interest and skill than usual, each year group had one or two 'outlaws', so to speak. This year was no different. Such outlaws would continually test the system, subtly defying ancient departmental policies. Given the slightest opportunity, they would waste no time exploiting any situation that allowed for mischief making.

The topic of this anatomy tutorial was the genital system of large mammals. While the lecturer was enthusiastic, he made no allowance for the fact that it was Friday afternoon. His students were more interested in getting the weekend off to a fine start in the pub. Malcolm was the only one in the room keen to get this practical anatomy session underway. Mr Pienaar's monotonous tone was, almost literally, a killer; dulling the senses, sending students into a deep comatose state.

Malcolm, however, was wearing his menacing grin that exposed his teeth and drew back his cheeks, making him look like a close relative of Beelzebub! He made sure he had the donkey specimen, and set about the task of dissecting it with surprising glee. The idea was to dissect and learn about the urological system including, among other things, the animal's kidneys, testicles and penile organ.

Malcolm dedicated the whole afternoon to dissecting the donkey's penis. At seventy five centimetres long, with a circumference of fourteen centimetres, a fine-sized specimen it was too. You could have played baseball with it if you were so inclined! He was meticulous in his work, taking the utmost care with each incision. Michelangelo would have been proud of that particular display of workmanship. At the end of the tutorial, while the other students obediently returned the tissue samples to the formaldehyde storage vessels, Malcolm secretly placed the dissected organ into some ice he had hidden in his bag.

After the session, he made an unusual stop at his brother's General Practitioner surgery to pick up a urine catheter and bag. He then purchased three litres of pineapple juice, before going home. That night, Malcolm carefully inserted and stitched the catheter into the donkey's penile organ before putting the revised organ into the deep freeze. The urine bag he filled with pineapple juice.

There was a great deal of noise and jostling at half-time, thousands of spectators making their way to the toilets. Malcolm had to queue for several minutes before he had the opportunity to squeeze through the compact human wall formed by men standing shoulder to shoulder at the urinals.

He found a space, quickly unzipped his fly, and hauled out the huge donkey organ, holding it in both hands. Eyes widened around him as he took a step back to avoid coming into contact with the stainless steel urinal. He squeezed his thighs together, causing a stream of 'urine' to gush forth, as if squirted from a garden hose. It sounded like hail stones falling on a tin roof, splattering wet the floor for quite a distance. Struggling to keep a straight face as jaws dropped around him, Malcolm started to whistle a cheery tune as he went about his business. The man standing to his left almost choked with disbelief, staring first at the organ, then at Malcolm then back to the organ.

Along the line of men, heads rotated to get a glimpse of this monstrosity of a member. Shoes were wet due to a concentration lapse of those standing in the line. Conversation dried up, as people stood on tiptoe to get a visual confirmation of the rumour going around the room.

After a few minutes, the stream began to dwindle. Malcolm gave the organ a good few smacks against the urinal to shake off the last few drops. The thuds were probably heard in the car park. Tucking it back into his trousers, he turned to face the stunned crowd. He gave the man closest to him a smirk, and said jauntily, "I needed that!" before striding out. The still silent crowd parted like the Red Sea for Moses. Malcolm was impressed when a fan stood to attention and saluted him, as he departed with a confident air.

Tobacco Pouch

"One day, the evil you inflict will come back to haunt you!" This story proves it.

Peter Magi was one of those people with no respect for the law or any other type of authority, so it follows that he would have no respect for the dead either.

At the beginning of his medical career, Peter attended a dissection class that dealt with dissection of the thorax. He took it upon himself to remove the skin over the breast of the cadaver that had been assigned to him. Ignoring the rules, he took the tissue home. He decided to use it to make a tobacco pouch, using fishing twine to close the edges, and a purse string to open and close the completed pouch.

Thereafter, he filled it with tobacco. He delighted in showing off to his fellow male students by producing the pouch, and proceeding to use the tobacco within to roll himself a smoke. He took great care to ensure that there were no faculty members in the vicinity when he did so.

His chickens came home to roost some years later. After completion of the pre-graduate training, Peter had drifted into the field of specialisation. He was still a very new registrar within the post-graduate department, and got on quite well with Professor Willis. After giving an in-depth speech about the controversy surrounding laparoscopic surgery in pregnant women, the Professor invited Peter to join him for a drink.

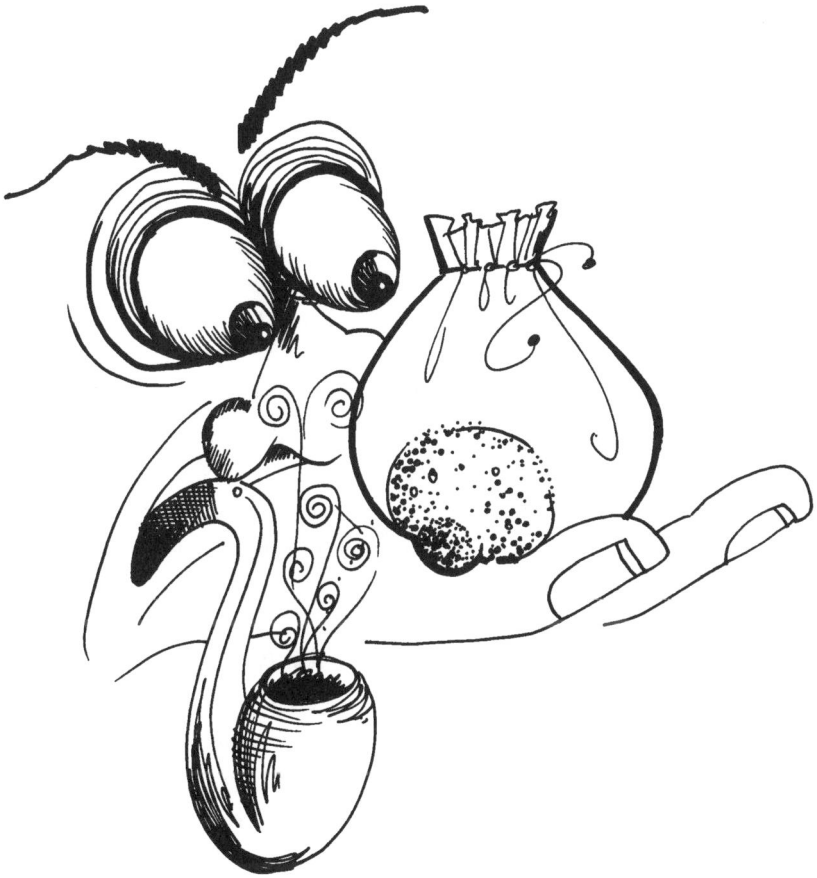

The professor enjoyed a smoke and offered Peter his packet of cigarettes. Declining, Peter reached into his pocket and pulled out his tobacco pouch, placing it on the desk in front of him, and began to roll pinches of tobacco into his cigarette paper.

The Professor looked at the pouch in bewilderment. "What is that?" he asked with an uncomfortable chuckle.

Peter began to laugh himself, and explained: "Just a stupid phase I went through during dissection..."

That statement cost him his career.

The Bill

Jon Megan is a successful property developer with an impressive passive income. He owns property all over the world, and more luxury cars than you could shake a stick at. Despite his great wealth, Jon was tighter than a duck's arse; he never spent more than he really had to. As for tipping – forget it! His jeans and Hawaiian shirts (bought back in the eighties, when Miami Vice was cool) did nothing to hint at the man's wealth. He didn't wear any big name labels, and had never hankered after a Rolex watch.

Jon was enjoying yet another holiday in the Seychelles, when he took quite a tumble during a water-skiing session, putting his back out. Back home in the States, he put up with the pain for a month before a friend recommended a chiropractor...in London. No problem. Jon arranged some business in London, and was at the Primrose Hill Street Clinic within the week.

Rail Jacobs is a chiropractor specialising in sports medicine. He had managed to build up a successful practice in five years. A good deal of his patients are word-of-mouth referrals. He took a lengthy medical history from Jon, concentrating on the aches and pains brought on by various sporting activities. When he was satisfied that he had all the information he needed, he engaged Jon in some personal small talk.

"So you're not from around here?" Jon's American accent had not fooled the ears of Rail Jacobs.
"No, I'm from the States. A friend of yours, Burt Niles, told me to come and see you," Jon answered.

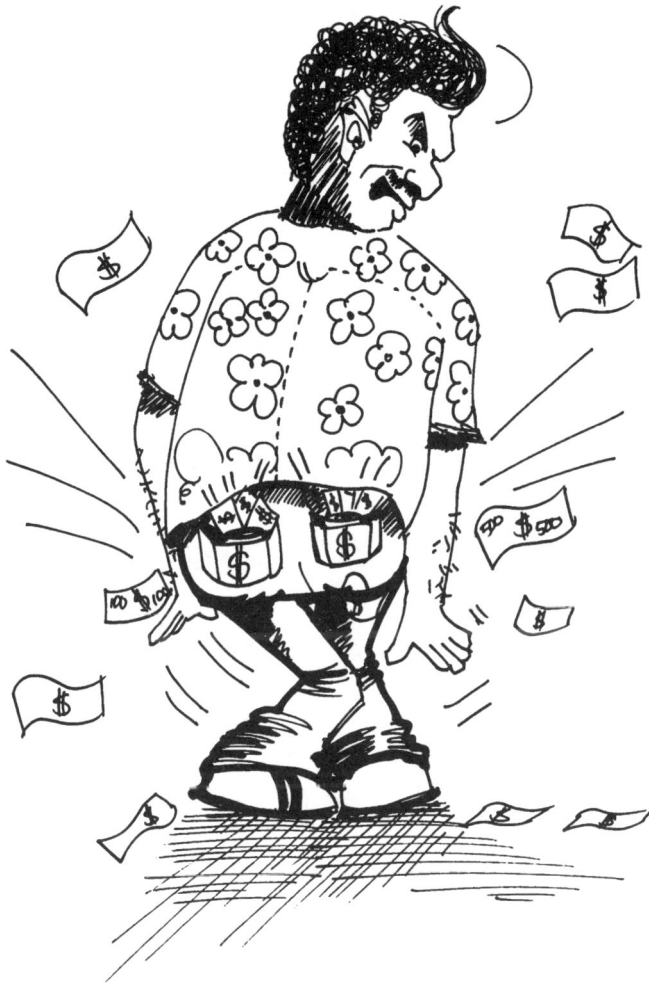

"Burt!" Rail exclaimed. "I haven't seen him for ages. How is he?"

"Very well. He still drinks like a fish, and has bought yet another yacht that he was showing off at the club!" Jon chuckled.

"I must give him a call," Rail muttered.

He was beginning to wonder what this scruffy Herbert was doing hanging around with the likes of Burt Niles. Jon had obviously spoken to Burt at the Yacht Club. They didn't let any old Tom, Dick or Harry onto the premises. He was still pondering this, when he told Jon to go to the treatment room and undress for the assessment and manipulation that was to follow.

Jon stripped to his undies and piled his clothes on a chair. He removed his bulging wallet from his trouser pocket and placed in on top of the pile. Rail entered the room and found Jon perched on the treatment table. As he began his examination of the patient, Rail couldn't help noticing the black leather Gucci wallet, almost bursting at the seams. As he continued to work, his eyes kept sliding off to look at the papers hanging out of the wallet. It was cash, not merely old receipts, which gave the wallet its fat appearance. Rail was bemused. How did such a scruff come to have so much money?

He did his best to concentrate on the treatment. When he finished, he left the room while Jon got dressed.
"So how much do I owe you?" Jon asked, as he walked back into the office.
Rail had to think fast. The current billing system allowed him to charge two hundred pounds for a first-time assessment and manipulation. This patient was clearly good for a lot more. He stalled. "How will you be paying?"
"Cash – if that's all right with you?" Jon raised his eyebrows.
Rail let out a nervous cough. "Cash works for me! That will be a thousand pounds then." He added quickly, "Good treatment doesn't come cheap!"
As Jon peeled off the notes, Rail decided that he was actually doing him a favour. Carrying that kind of weight around couldn't be good for a person.

When Jon left, Rail decided to give Burt a call to thank him for the referral.
"You're welcome – I hope you stung him for a few extra quid!" Burt laughed.
"Big time!" Rail confirmed. "How the hell did he get so much money?"

"What? I thought you knew. That is Jon Megan of Megan Properties. The guy is minted!" Burt couldn't believe his friend hadn't known this.

"So I could have charged him even more?" Rail was sensing a missed opportunity.

"A lot more!" Burt paused. "You've taught me something, Rail. The next time I visit any Doctor's office, I am going to make sure my wallet is tucked safely out of sight!"

Zebra

Adrian had the misfortune to be born into a family of racists. He grew up to believe that white people were superior to those with any other skin tone. It didn't occur to him to ask for any justification for this reasoning; he had simply learnt it from his family environment.

As he grew into an adult and entered the world of work, he began to notice that not everyone shared his belief in white superiority. His job in a plastics factory brought him into the company of people of other races. He soon learnt that his racist comments were not acceptable. He managed to be politically correct on the surface, but his ingrained bigotry remained. Fortunately, higher powers sometimes prevail, and life lessons are taught to those very much in need.

Adrian was in his usual position on the plastic moulding assembly, on the day that one of the manifold outlets ignited, releasing a spray of hot plastic solvent over a large area of the factory. Badly burnt, Adrian was rushed to hospital to receive immediate treatment for third degree burns, covering more than fifty percent of his body. His condition was serious, as the skin not only helps the body to retain moisture, but also provides a natural barrier against bacteria.

Since Adrian didn't have sufficient undamaged skin for the surgeons to harvest for grafting onto the burnt areas, a temporary graft was made from skin taken from a cadaver. It sounds gruesome, but it did the trick!

Adrian was anaesthetised before being hurried into theatre to receive his temporary protective layer. Patient recovery was

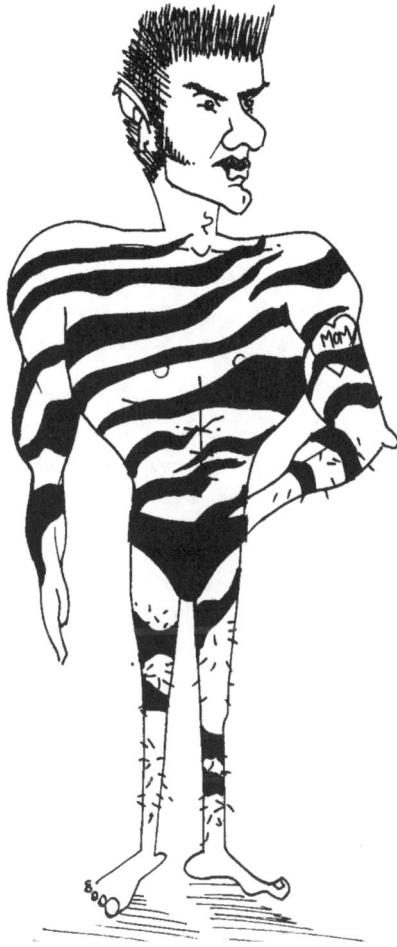

something to behold, when Adrian realised that the donor skin had come from a black African male. His pulse rate and pressure escalated as he glared at his black stripes. Given his discriminatory tendencies, it must have been quite an ordeal, as he struggled with the concept that the skin from a person of a supposedly inferior race was giving him the chance of survival.

To make matters worse, Adrian's body did not reject the cadaver skin. It became permanent, giving him and his family something to think about.

The Bite in the Bag

Paul Jan was working as a labourer on a horse farm near the town of Roberton. He was loading bales of hay from a storage shed, onto the back of a truck. The bales were tightly stacked in the shed. He cursed himself for leaving his work gloves at home. He shoved his hand between two bales, and started to wiggle one out. When he had made a bigger gap, he pushed his arm in further, trying to reach behind the bale so that he could pull it out. He suddenly heard a loud hiss and felt a sharp pain in his hand. He screamed, snatching his arm out of the gap, shocked to find a long snake dangling from his hand.

At the local clinic, Nic was enjoying an uneventful shift when Paul Jan rushed in. The security guards tried to stop him; so that they could check the rucksack he was carrying over his shoulder. Pale and sweaty, Paul Jan insisted on seeing a doctor, refusing to give up his rucksack for inspection. Nic told the guards that he would handle things, and waved Paul Jan into the examination room.

"What's the problem?" Nic asked.
Paul Jan explained that he had been bitten by a snake whilst moving bales of hay.
"When did this happen?"
"About an hour ago – I rushed straight here!"
"Did you get a good look at the snake?" Nic was trying to find out what kind of snake was involved, as there are three classifications of snakebite, and three different treatments. Snake venom can be neurotoxic - affecting the nervous system and breathing; cytotoxic – attacks the skin and tissue under the bite, sometimes spreading to affect entire limbs, or haemotoxic – attacks red blood cells, causing

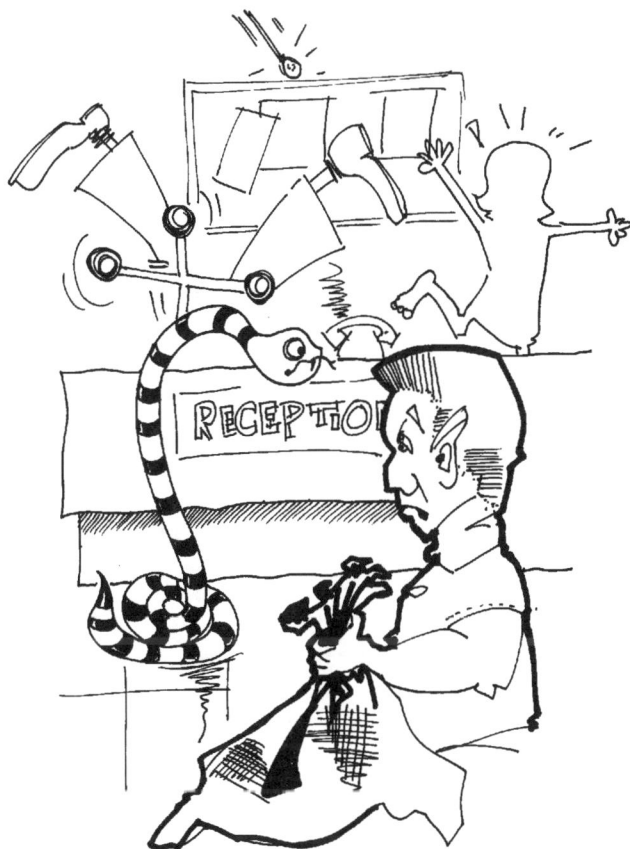

them to rupture within the vascular system.

"Yes, in fact I brought it with me...in the rucksack." Paul Jan twitched his head at the rucksack he still carried over his shoulder.

Nic was pleased. Betty the nurse sighed with impatience, wondering why the guy hadn't said so before.

"Come on then," Nic invited. "Pop it on the table. The sooner we identify it, the sooner we can treat you!"

"Well, if you're sure..." Paul Jan hesitated.

Betty tutted. "We have other patients waiting to see the doctor, Sir."

Grimacing, Paul Jan drew his hand out of the rucksack. Nic jumped back in alarm. Betty – no spring chicken – made an admirable leap onto a chair.

Despite having a good grip of its neck, Paul Jan couldn't stop the snake's furious writhing, spitting and hissing.

"It's alive?" A stupid question, but Nic was in a state of shock. He really hadn't expected the patient to pull a live snake out of his bag, in much the same way as a magician pulls a rabbit out of a hat.

The waiting room was chaotic with would-be patients scattering like frightened hens. Even those on crutches found some speed.

Recovering slightly as he watched Paul Jan shoved the snake back into the rucksack, Nic managed to admonish his patient, "You can not bring a live Cobra into a clinic!"

"Well, at least we know what it is now!" Paul Jan replied huffily.

Surprise Test

Five medical students shared digs. It took them two minutes by car to the academic's hospital car park, and another five minutes to walk through the hospital to the lecture rooms. So, on average, they would take about eight minutes to get from digs to a seat, just in time for a class.

The fifth year surgical block lectures went on for three long months. To make matters worse, Dr Cruz, an anal retentive surgical lecturer, enjoyed threatening late afternoon spot tests. The bastard.

At two o'clock one Friday afternoon, it was announced that we would be writing a spot test. Steynberg ran from the lecture room, brushed through the arriving stragglers, and made for the public phone in the hall. Back at the digs, Goose and Kaps had decided to cut class, beginning the weekend festivities early. One frantic phone call put an end to their plans.

"Test! Test! We've got a spot test!" Steynberg shouted, before slamming the phone down, and racing back to class. Goose and Kaps put aside their preparations for the long weekend, and dashed into class just in time to take the test.

Naturally, they were greatly indebted to Steynberg for the timely warning.

A few weeks later, the final lecture of the day was cancelled. The lads found themselves at a bit of a loose end. Strolling back to the digs, Goose, Kaps and Steynberg got to wondering where Snails was.

Of the four students, Snails was the closest to an introvert. He was an odd character, occasionally displaying flashes of genius, always picking a new and short-lived fad. One month it might be brandy tasting, the next he'd have taken up photography.

"I bet he's asleep!" said Kaps. The three lads were simultaneously afflicted with an evil grin. They made their way back to the hospital foyer, where they could look through the sliding doors at the entrance, across the car park, and straight down Dodge Street. Their house was towards the bottom end of Dodge Street. Goose dropped a coin into the public phone box and dialled. "Uargh. Hello? Hello?" a sleepy voice answered.

"Snails! Test! Test! Test!" Goose bellowed and slammed down the phone.

The lads eagerly watched Dodge Street. They weren't disappointed. A white Beetle suddenly reversed into the street and sped up the road towards the hospital. It roared into the car park, almost taking out a couple of pensioners who found they weren't as nimble as they used to be. Snails parked in the ambulance zone and sprang from the car, dropping books and papers all over. It was a sight to behold. At the best of times Snails didn't move with the grace of an athlete. Watching him hop, skip and jump at speed, whilst attempting to keep his sandals from falling off, was more than his audience could bear. As Snails sped into the foyer, hot and sweaty with panic, he was ever so slightly confused to be greeted by shrieks of laughter.

At last the penny dropped. "You bloody skanks!"

The Relative

Few first world inhabitants have had the misfortune to experience a South African public Accident and Emergency unit, where evenings and weekends are associated with alcohol and drug abuse and the barbaric acts of violence that may follow.

The unit comprises of two sections, divided by steel bars. The waiting area is filled with rows of stained and tatty wooden seats. The floor is stained with blood and other unsavoury secretions. People spend hours sitting around, waiting for treatment for themselves or for family and friends. Security personnel stand guard at the entrance gate leading to the treatment area, controlling the influx of patients and barring entry to the gangs outside when they come to finish off a victim. Only brutally maimed patients are admitted through the gates without a security interrogation session.

On a winter evening in July, the casualty unit was packed to capacity with people listening to monotonous drunken arguments from outside, and the groans from the treatment cubicles filtered into the waiting area.

Suddenly all the noise seemed to cease, and a number of people shuffled out of the waiting area. I watched carefully as two men approached the security gate. They were of the same build and complexion, and stood close together. Their staggering gaits left me in no doubt that they had been drinking heavily. To my horror, I noticed that one of the men had an axe lodged in the side of his head, the handle pressed tightly against his shoulder. Fresh blood was still seeping out of the wound, staining his creased shirt.

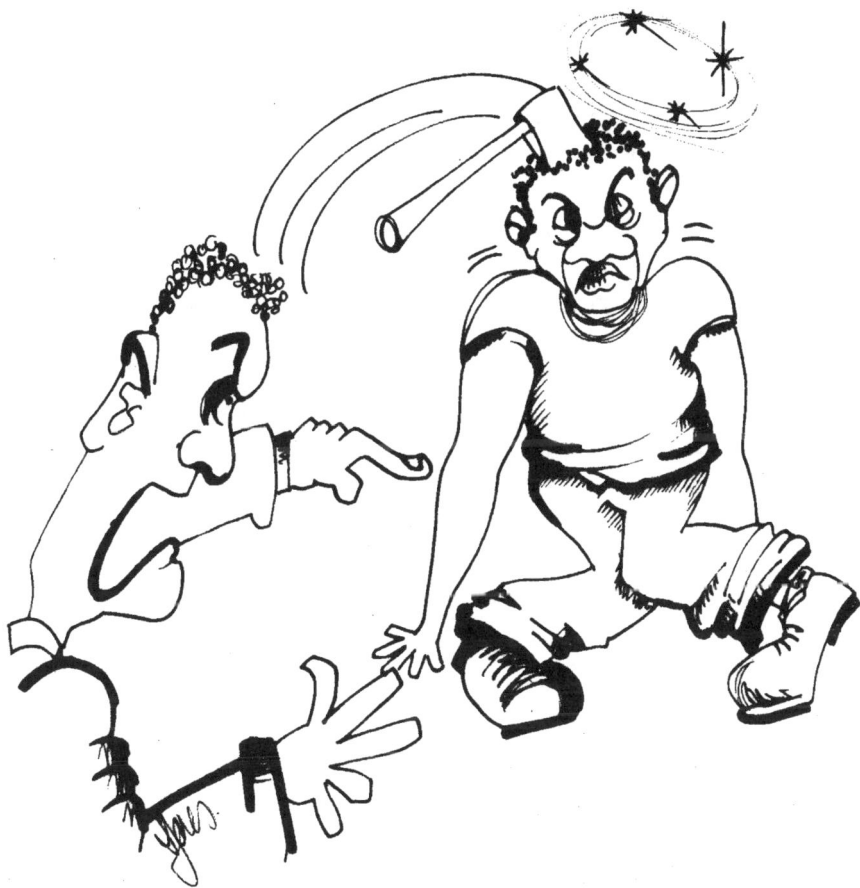

I nodded to the security guard. He opened the gate without hesitation, leading the patient and, I presumed, his relative into the treatment area. It struck me as odd that whilst most people shy away from gruesome injuries, the man's relative just seemed rather despondent, almost if he had lost something. He kept his eyes fixed on the axe. Wherever the patient walked, he followed closely behind.

From a clinical point of view, the obvious course of action was to determine whether the axe blade had penetrated the cranium; and if so, to what extent. I instructed a cranium X-ray, followed by a CT scan be done. Once again the relative displayed the oddest behaviour. He was quite literally the patient's shadow.

The men arrived back in the treatment area. As the resident casualty officer, I took it upon myself to take a patient history, and decided to get some background from the patient's relative. I began by asking him his name, address and contact numbers. The bizarre truth emerged when I asked him how he was related to the patient.

He frowned at me, looked almost offended and declared, "I'm his neighbour. The sight of him makes me absolutely sick!"
Taken aback, I continued my questioning and was rewarded with the following information: The neighbours had had an argument over a sack of fermenting wine, that the patient had been delighted to find buried under a tyre in his back yard. As it was the weekend, he took full advantage of his good fortune, consuming the beverage. Such was his thirst for the hooch, that he didn't take the precaution of smuggling it into the privacy of his house. His neighbour had also had more than adequate refreshment from another sack of hooch, and was livid when he spotted the patient partaking of the hooch that he had hidden under the tyre for safe keeping.

Unfortunately for the patient, the axe had been close at hand when his neighbour had decided to put a stop to his carry on. As the patient bent his head to suck at the sack, his neighbour crept up behind him, and swung with the axe.

It is important to understand that in African culture the axe is an important tool used in everyday life. During winter months, it becomes an absolute necessity to provide wood for fuel. It is not so surprising that the neighbour was not about to let the axe out of his sight. If that meant accompanying the patient to the A and E to await its removal, then so be it!

Suspect Renal Nurse

Renal failure is an unfortunate consequence of various acute and chronic illnesses. When the kidneys and their filtering tubes are functioning insufficiently, toxins and other biochemical abnormalities begin to accumulate in the blood. These imbalances can have profound symptomatic effects on patients, including energy loss, fluid retention and in severe cases, cardiac arrest.

Many people undergo renal dialysis (where a machine filters the blood) on a temporary basis, while they wait for a kidney transplant. For some, it becomes a permanent solution. Those receiving long-term dialysis need to provide continuous access to a vein for every treatment. These may be once or twice a week, maybe more, depending on kidney function, to allow the operator to rig them up to the dialysis machine.

In order to minimise discomfort, doctors have created a unique surgical procedure, called a venous-arterio fistula. A surgeon makes a small incision in the forearm, and uses tiny stitches to join an artery and vein. This creates a dilated and pressurised blood reservoir, which is easily accessible when the patient needs to be connected to the dialysis machine.

Mary Jones decided to give up her retail job in favour of training to be a nurse. She became a nursing assistant, and had high hopes of progressing up the ranks as she completed each training phase. The practical side of nursing means that new recruits are introduced to patients very early on in their careers. Although this seems justified in

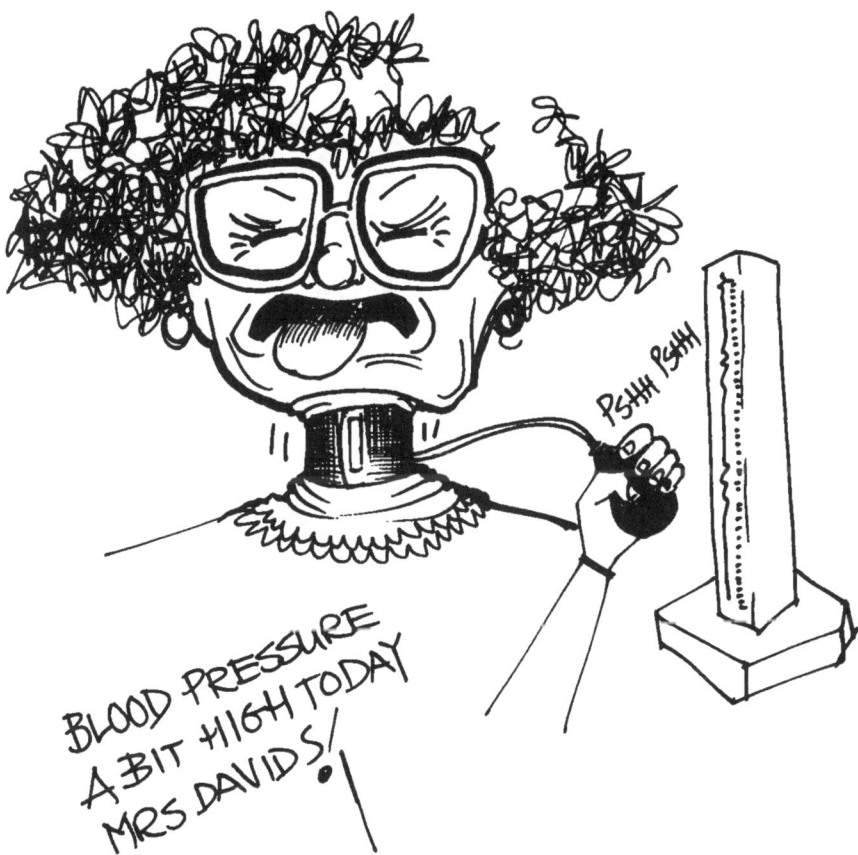

BLOOD PRESSURE
A BIT HIGH TODAY
MRS DAVIDS!

PSHH PSHH

a clinical multi-disciplinary environment, on rare occasions, it has the potential to backfire!

One morning, the nursing superiors had lectured Mary on the use of the blood pressure monitoring equipment, and how the arteries in a patient's arm give the blood pressure as the cuff is deflated. Mary was quietly confident that she could differentiate between the various components: cuff, tubing and the machine itself. She had had her own blood pressure checked by her GP often enough – how hard could it be?

Lily was the Charge Nurse of the Renal Dialysis Suite that day. Due to two staff nurses calling in sick, she found herself with some extra nursing assistants. Now she had rookie nurses to keep an eye on, as well as the seven patients. "I don't want to see any of you taking blood pressures from the same arm as the surgical fistulas, otherwise Dr Goldberg will have *my* neck!" she warned the rookies.

Granny Davids had a long history of kidney problems, probably stemming from her diabetes. Her age and other systemic complications ruled out a transplant; so the poor old dear was dependant on weekly kidney filtration. All the dialysis meant that venous access was problematic, so surgeons were forced to create a fistula on both her forearms.

As Mary entered Granny Davids' cubicle, she pulled the curtains closed to preserve the patient's dignity. Ironically, this act of kindness might have been the undoing of both patient and nursing assistant. "Good afternoon, Mrs Davids. How are you today?" Mary greeted her patient.
"Ooh my dear, I'm feeling so poorly today!" came the querulous reply.
"Don't you worry," Mary assured the granny. "We'll finish you off today...I mean, I'll take good care of you!"

A quick check of Granny Davids' arms revealed a fistula on each. Remembering Lily's earlier instructions, Mary stuck her head through the curtains, and was informed by a colleague that Lily had stepped out of the suite for a moment. Hmm. Artery and cuff. Never use limbs with fistulas. Mary put two and two together, and decided to use her initiative.

Not much later, Lily peered through the curtains. "Stop!" she yelled, horrified. The machine was still inflating, as Granny Davids was being throttled by the blood pressure cuff around her neck. The veins on her neck stood out and her eyes bulged. Her face and ears nicely complemented her blue-rinsed hair. Mary was waiting patiently for the digital blood pressure reading, while Granny Davids' head began to sway from side to side. Of course, the fact that she had stopped breathing at this stage, may have contributed to her general apathy.

Lily arrived in the nick of time, and Mary was relegated to bedpan duty.

The Press Incident

A bus carrying passengers to work lost control and veered off the road. It overturned, leaving twenty people injured. The District Hospital of Port Nolan was put on alert, and the big city hospital, a few hours' drive away, was contacted for assistance. The first paramedics on the scene reported that their triage evaluation concluded three critically injured patients; conscious, but with severe neck and head injuries. These patients were airlifted to the major hospital for specialist scans, neurosurgery, orthopaedic and intensive care support.

The police closed the road temporarily. Local radio stations were requested to inform road users to find alternative routes. Then the media got wind of the situation. Before long, the hospital entrance was awash with reporters and their camera crews; demanding information, hoping for a good picture for the front page.

Inside, the Accident and Emergency department was in a chaotic state: patients on beds, trolleys, chairs, crutches and, when all else failed, the floor. The place was littered with bloodstained swabs, drip sets and papers. The double swing doors separated the madness inside from that outside.

Jake and Reuben worked tirelessly, sifting through the injured, referring patients to the necessary departments, organising relevant tests for the patients who required them. The last thing they needed was any aggravation from stragglers left over from the night before.

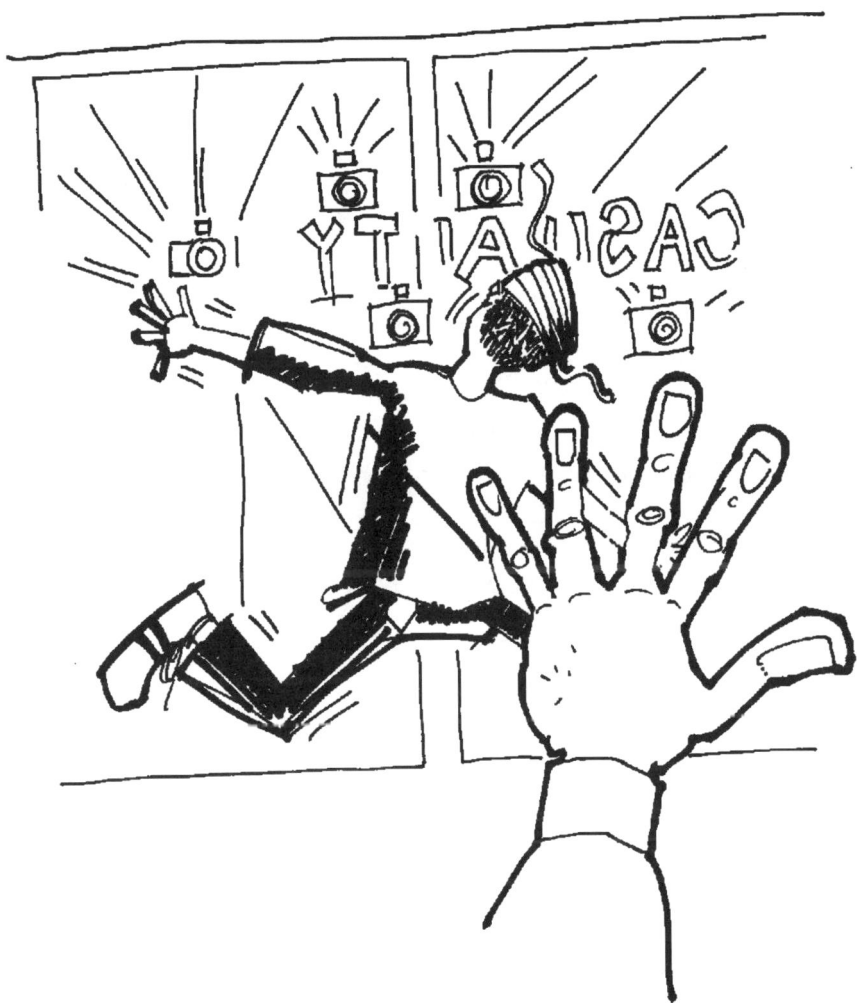

Peter Mohan had been admitted, inebriated, a few hours previously. The regular binge drinker had been involved in a punch-up at the local bar, and had suffered a nasty head wound. The main superficial temporal artery over the temple head area had been severed, and bled profusely. Jake needed Peter to keep still while he deep-sutured the wound, but Peter had not been very cooperative. The wound was packed with a pressure dressing, which made Peter look like a *mummy* with two moving nystagmus eyes, visible through the slits. When news came in of the bus accident, Jake moved Peter into a side room next to casualty, hoping he'd sleep the booze off.

Reuben was working diligently at his desk, making the required notes and sketches of the injuries suffered by passengers on the bus. This is an essential task, as it covers doctors in the event of any future medico-legal issues. Peter woke up and staggered towards Reuben, shouting incoherently. Reuben suffered a sense of humour failure, and snapped at Peter to get back to his bed. Ignoring the advice of his doctor, Peter began to unwind his bandage, causing his wound to start bleeding again. He lurched over Reuben's desk, dripping blood everywhere. Fear of contaminated blood, and a build up of anger led to Reuben's transformation from professional health worker, to monster-doctor with super-human strength.

He jumped up from the desk and grabbed Peter by the collar and belt and, holding him like a battering ram, ran towards the doors, bandages flapping. As Peter's head burst through the doors, Reuben let go. The *momentum* kept Peter airborne, just long enough for him to scatter reporters on the ground. With the doctor's words, "Now get the hell out of here!" ringing in their ears, the reporters got both their quote and a fabulous front-page picture.

As he let Peter fly through the air, Reuben was lit up by the camera flashes that caught him. He realised that there was no going back. Some legal aid was going to come in handy!

Withdrawal Junkie

Alcohol abuse is a global problem, affecting all levels of society. It can be a contributing factor to violent crime, motor vehicle accidents and domestic problems. It may present itself as continual drinking over a period of time, or as periodic binge drinking. It is characterised by the inability to stop drinking during these periods. These situations are often associated with mood disorders such as stress and depression.

Alcohol withdrawal syndrome is a side effect affecting heavy drinkers who suddenly stop drinking. It may involve mild symptoms of sickness, blurred vision, mental confusion, delirium tremors (the DTs) right through to life-threatening seizures.

Pete Roux was known to his Community Hospital as a heavy drinker. He worked as a grape-picker in the wine region where the hospital was situated. Every now and then, the owner of the wine farm would give his staff litres of the excess wine that didn't get bottled. Naturally, this would lead to Pete and his co-workers indulging in a bout of binge drinking.

Bed space in the Community Hospital was restricted on the morning that Pete was admitted, having been diagnosed with Alcohol Withdrawal Syndrome. He showed early signs of the DTs and mental confusion. Dr Sam Goldberg, a young resident casualty officer, decided to keep him in for further investigation and treatment. This decision was prudent, as it is important to rule out other problems with symptoms that may mimic the DTs, such as diabetes or head

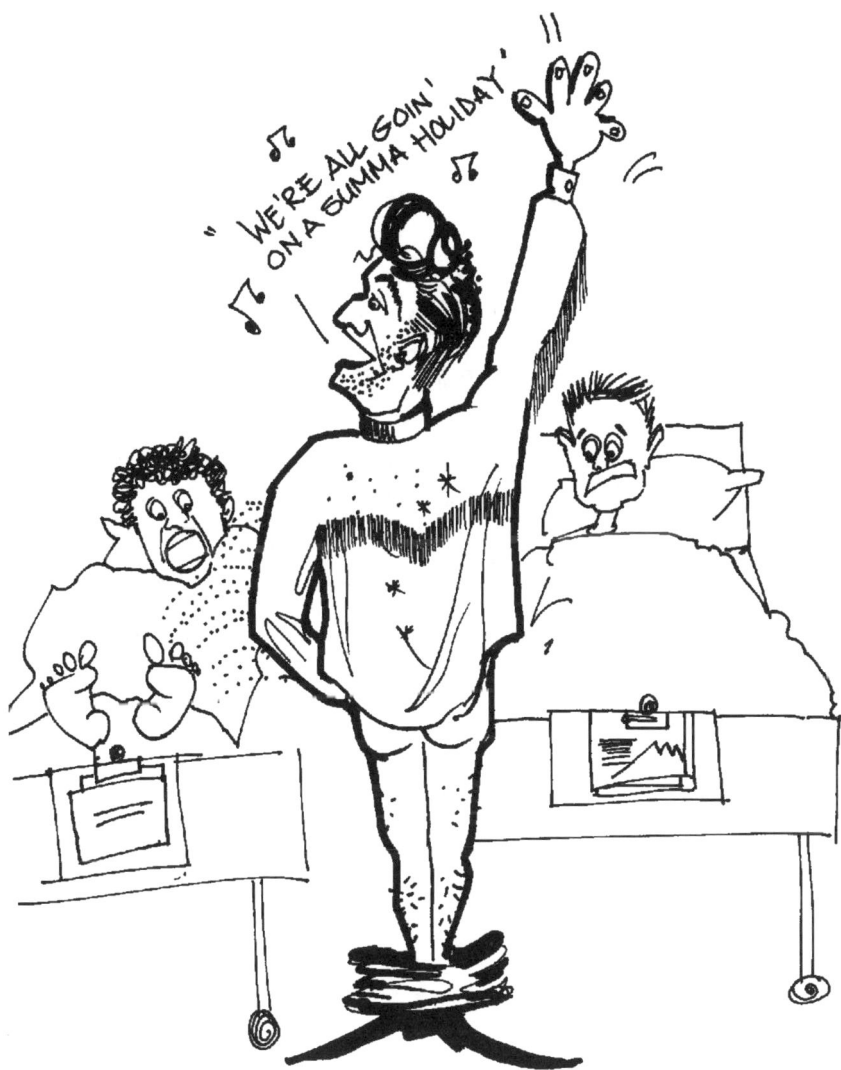

injuries. The treatment regime of intravenous benzodiazepines has potential side effects, also warranting in-hospital monitoring.

With the hospital almost full, Sam had no choice but to allocate Pete a bed in the casualty ward, between Mrs Simone Beukers and Mr Piet Skeupers. The ward measured approximately ten by fifteen metres, with five examination cubicles on the left-hand side and a Plaster of Paris cubicle in the bottom right-hand corner. Sam's desk was slap-bang in the middle.

The curtains were drawn around each cubicle. It wasn't long before yelling was heard from behind one set of curtains. Sam rushed in, to find Pete urinating on Simone, whilst giving an ear-splitting rendition of Cliff Richard's "Summer Holiday". He did his best to convince Pete to settle down, and opted to sedate him with a powerful anxiolytic drug. Unfortunately, even the maximum dose did nothing to shut Pete up. He became more blasphemous and abusive to all around him. By that stage, Simone needed something to calm her nerves. The nurses were demanding more action from the beleaguered Sam.

Help arrived in the form of Duncan Renforth, a sprightly doctor of the old-school who had worked at the hospital, on and off, for over forty-five years. He was in a league if his own, as he didn't fall under the jurisdiction of any authority or medical guidance directives. At the ripe old age of seventy-seven, Duncan did not require anyone's advice. He believed that all politicians were fascists, with no role to play in the health service or any matters concerning it.

Marching to the suture cupboard, Duncan ripped out a package and disappeared behind the curtains. Some shouting could be heard, but it was quickly followed by a long groan, and then silence. Whisking back the curtains, he emerged looking very pleased with himself. Pete lay in the bed – very much subdued - with the blanket up to his chin.

Strolling past the interviewing station, Duncan smiled. "Don't worry, he won't disturb you again. I'll see him in the morning." Sam glanced over at Pete. He lay perfectly still with his eyes staring straight ahead. Nurses helped Simone and Piet get cleaned up and back into bed. Everyone wondered what Duncan had done behind the curtains.

At nine o'clock the next morning, Duncan arrived and requested a stitch-cutter. Sam rushed to Pete's bedside with the required implement; eager to see what would happen next. As Duncan approached the bed, Pete glared at him and started to tremble.

"Oh come now!" Duncan chided him. "Don't tell me you're still holding a grudge!"

Sam couldn't believe his eyes when Duncan threw back the blanket. Pete's scrotum was stitched, very neatly, to the mattress! No wonder he hadn't moved all night.